Drugs in Conception, Pregnancy and Childbirth

Judy Priest trained as an anthropologist and a nurse, and has worked in Britain, the United States and West Africa. For ten years she taught couples to prepare for their baby's birth and the months that follow and trained antenatal teachers for the National Childbirth Trust. She ran workshops for health professionals in antenatal education throughout the UK. She is the editor of *The Baby Annual*, she lives in Oxford with her husband and three children. She currently works in education.

A project like this book rests on the help and support of so many people. I am grateful to all the parents who have shared their stories, described their dilemmas and trusted me to use their words and experiences. Individual people also helped. Judith Schott read many chapters with her characteristic thoroughness, and Veronica Taylor listened when the going got tough. Christine Tompson shared her work on induction when I needed a new view. My NCT students told me stories and asked good questions. I thank them all. But above all, I am grateful to my children, Freya, Russell, and Daniel, who accepted the disruption and inconvenience of living with this book for a year and a half. My husband read chunks of the manuscript carefully and critically yet never faltered in his encouragement. Best of all, he simply picked up the daily tasks I ignored so I could finish the project. Thanks, Tony.

Drugs in Conception, Pregnancy and Childbirth

Judy Priest

with Kathy Attawall

Thorsons

An Imprint of HarperCollins*Publishers*

While the creators of this work have made every effort to ensure that the information presented is as accurate and up-to-date as possible at the time of publication, medical and pharmaceutical knowledge is constantly changing and the application of it to particular circumstances depends on many factors. Therefore readers are urged always to consult a qualified medical specialist for individual advice. This book should not be used as an alternative to appropriate medical care. The author and publishers cannot be held liable for any errors and omissions, or actions that may be taken as a result of using it.

Thorsons
An Imprint of HarperCollins*Publishers*
77–85 Fulham Palace Road,
Hammersmith, London W6 8JB

First published by Pandora Press 1990
This edition 1996

Published by Thorsons 1997
1 3 5 7 9 10 8 6 4 2

A catalogue record for this book
is available from the British Library

ISBN 0 7225 3594 5

Printed and bound in Great Britain

Contents

Foreword

In pregnancy women are told that they must do everything they can to make the baby 100 per cent perfect – to watch their diet, and avoid all drugs and cigarettes and alcohol. It is implied that if a woman is casual about what she eats or drinks, if she smokes, takes aspirin to relieve a headache, for example, or even has the occasional glass of wine, she has only herself to blame if her baby is not perfect. When a woman has done any of these things, perhaps even before she knew she was pregnant, she may go through the whole of the rest of her pregnancy believing that she has harmed her baby.

We may think that today we have set aside the superstitions and rituals of less sophisticated cultures. Yet the western way of birth has created its own rituals and taboos. Rules about pregnant women's behaviour have become as rigid as in any Third World society, where women are careful never to step over a donkey's tethering rope in case the umbilical cord gets twisted round the baby's neck. Surrounded by dangers, the modern pregnant woman tries to pick her way, as if on stepping stones at the edge of a precipice, to the goal of a healthy baby.

This whole approach to pregnancy is dangerously simplistic. The perils by which we are surrounded cannot be a woman's sole responsibility. Toxic fumes belched by factories, pesticides, polluted air – try as women may to avoid these dangers, it is beyond their power to do so. It is no longer a question of individual or even local responsibilities. Most of these dangers can only be dealt with at an international or national level.

Another result of imposing on mothers a burden of personal responsibility for anything and everything that happens to the developing fetus is that the *social* context within which pregnancy and birth take place is ignored. Instead of looking at how real women's lives are lived, and the pressures and stresses with which they have to cope, pregnant women are told they must avoid all potential risks. In practice, this is impossible. For it is usually not a matter of choosing between an action or substance that is dangerous and another that is harmless, but of *balancing risks*.

We know, for example, that pregnant women should not smoke. It deprives the unborn baby of oxygen, exposing it to the risks of intrauterine growth retardation and premature birth. But a woman who smokes may be doing so because it is the only way she knows of shaping her day, making a space for herself, taking time to relax, or talking with co-workers. If she lives in a high-rise flat with three children under five, it may give her a moment of illusory peace so that she does not let rip and hit the children. She knows that she ought not to smoke, but, without perhaps being at all aware of it, she is balancing the risk of lashing out with violence against her children and introducing possible damage to the unborn baby inside her.

Risk assessment is important for all of us, whether or not we are expecting a baby. We have to be able to balance risks and quickly come to some kind of working decision, even though we may change our minds later, simply to be able to step into a road on which traffic is hurtling past. Parents are constantly having to do rapid risk assessments and make decisions. It is impossible to bring up a child without taking risks.

Concentrated focus on risk can be so terrifying that we become virtually paralysed, and construct a straitjacket of rigid rules and prohibitions to try and contain the dangers all around us. This is what western culture has tended to do to pregnant women.

There is an alternative. We can find out how to get the information we need in order to assess risks in the context of our own lives and relationships, our own needs and values.

This book contains a great deal of carefully investigated information about drugs in pregnancy and childbirth. But the reader will find no rules and regulations, no strictures about what she ought to do. The decisions are left to her and in some circumstances she may have to make difficult choices. A pregnant woman, for example, can never know exactly how she is going to feel during labour or what help she may need. Her best course of action is to be positive, realistic and flexible, and to be actively involved in all decisions made by those caring for her. This entails being able to make an informed assessment of the benefits and risks of obstetric interventions and different drugs. This book is the only place I know where women can get the facts about drugs in pregnancy and childbirth.

Judy Priest helps readers examine the mass of information and misinformation about drugs in pregnancy and birth, and has done meticulous and painstaking research into the enormously complicated subject of known and hypothetical damaging effects of many different kinds of medication, as well as the effects of different drugs on the baby and mother during labour. Her writing is deft, vivid and refreshingly down-to-earth. Yet right through these pages she tackles an even more vital question: how can we make choices between alternatives? How can we come to *any* decisions in a world of uncertainty?

Because there are much wider social implications in everything she says, she presents a powerful challenge to us all.

Sheila Kitzinger

How to Use This Book

Childbirth has never been safer for mothers or babies, yet we have never seemed so concerned with risk. We do not, by and large, spread our concern equally between the two people sharing the experience of pregnancy and birth: the woman and her baby. Worries about the mother's health are much less than they were a decade or two ago and minute compared to what they were a century ago (or what they still are in developing countries). Smaller families, better nutrition, public sanitation and sophisticated obstetric interventions have resulted in maternal mortality figures that are very, very small. Western women expect to be able to cope with the physical changes of pregnancy and the rigours of childbirth. They may still wake in the night and wonder, 'What is something awful happens to me ...' but the question is speculation rather than contingency planning, as would have been the case for their Victorian sisters.

The same cannot be said for women's feelings about the health and wellbeing of their babies. In the last few years, the worry has become so powerful that it warrants a label: 'reproductive anxiety'. Not surprisingly, the word comes from the United States where doctors get ahead by 'discovering' new syndromes and then publishing papers about them. It seems generally agreed that reproduction anxiety (probably soon to be known as RA in line with the penchant for initials that bedevils the medical profession!) is growing year by year. Norma Swenson, president of the Boston Women's Health

Collection said, 'I've worked with pregnant women for twenty years and there were always ones who seemed unduly agitated that something could go wrong. But they were the exceptions. Today, it seems the other way around. And I think that's sad.'

'Sad' perhaps, but hardly surprising when you consider what the media has served up for pregnant women in recent years. There were stories about infected paté and soft cheese causing listeriosis in developing babies – 26 babies died in 1988 in Britain. Then came warnings that vulnerable groups should be wary of salmonella in eggs and not to eat liver. Soon after, women's magazines warned pregnant women not to change the cat litter lest they pick up the organism that causes toxoplasmosis, a mild illness that can mean handicap or death for a growing baby. American women have been given advice warning them to avoid caffeine completely. And there are stories of bringing other people's pain into your livingroom: a breakfast television feature about the American woman suing a whisky company because the bottle-a-day she drank in pregnancy didn't have a warning label that said her son might be born mentally retarded, but he was. Every month brings a new story and a new worry – no wonder women are anxious.

It is as if being pregnant is like swimming in a sea full of sharks for some women. If they relax their guard for even a minute, they might be bitten, so they stay alert, gather ever greater amounts of information, and try and keep terrible things at bay.

One of the perceived 'sharks' is drugs. I began to wonder if the anxiety I was picking up from pregnant women about drugs was fact or fantasy. What were the real risks for mothers and babies? What drugs should they be concerned about, and what do we mean by drugs? What was the price of hypervigilence? Does being so anxious inhibit mothers and doctors from making good decisions? This last question may never be answered, but anxiety is certainly not good for the mother or the baby and it was also soon clear to me that hypervigilence leads women and doctors to some surprising decisions where drugs are concerned. Take this one, for instance: someone told me about a woman who broke her ribs when she was four months pregnant . She was denied pain relief and spent weeks in pain – it hurt every time she breathed. A non-pregnant woman treated in this way would have grounds for a legal suit for gross negligence. How had the doctor arrived at this decision and why did the woman herself accept it? What were the long-term consequences? The search was on for the answers – and the ultimate result is this book.

*   *   *

This looks like a book about drugs, but it is actually a book about making decisions about drugs. I wrote it because most of the help and advice currently on offer to pregnant women from lay and medical sources makes it harder, not easier, to make good decisions. Most advice about drugs is over-simplified ('Avoid all drugs'/'Don't drink'). Some is dogmatic and preachy ('Pain relief for labour spoils the experience') and a surprising amount is just plain wrong ('Don't bother giving up smoking if you haven't done so by the 16th week').

Here's a typical example, taken from *You and your Pregnancy* published by the British Medical Association. It deals with the issue of drugs in pregnancy under the heading 'Beware of Pills.' The author cautions 'It is a good idea now to take no drugs in early pregnancy' ('drugs' are not defined and we are not told what 'early pregnancy' is). Further down the paragraph, the author reminds the reader to 'beware not to poison the baby with nicotine from cigarettes or with alcohol or with drugs or any other dangerous substance.'

The trouble with that brief, unambiguous advice like this, echoed in nearly every book written for pregnant women, is that it disregards the complexity of our lives. For example, it presumes that women will know they are pregnant from the moment they are, and we know that's not so. It overlooks the fact that you may be addicted to tobacco or living in a world in which alcohol or use of illegal or 'street' drugs is an integral part of your life. You may have a chronic condition which requires drug therapy and will continue to need treatment during pregnancy.

What would be more helpful is some idea of how to weigh up the risks and benefits of a particular drug for you and your baby. The advice already cited gives no hint of this balancing act: it lumps drugs which have benefits, as well as risks, with things that are simply harmful, like smoking. And it gives no hint about the feelings behind such decisions. Reading the booklet would not help any of these women:

Jill is 14 weeks pregnant and has bronchitis. She feels rotten, has a temperature of 101° and has been in bed all day coughing. But she remembers reading in the booklet she picked up at a clinic that one shouldn't take drugs when pregnant, so she doesn't. Is that the best choice for Jill?
   Probably not.

And Anne worries. She takes medication every day to control her epilepsy. Now she wants to start a family but she knows that by taking those pills, she risks harming a developing baby. So she pushes the whole issue to the back of her mind. Is that the best choice?
   Probably not.

Most drug decisions are complex ones like this; they need more than a brisk exhortation or few sentences of factual information. They deserve a book of their own.

I have addressed this book to the pregnant woman herself. I know that many women will discuss these matters with their partners and some people who read it will not be pregnant women. But the central person in the decision is the woman who is contemplating pregnancy. She is carrying the baby and she is experiencing labour. To that woman I say, 'The final choice is yours', though others are probably deeply concerned with these matters, too.
   I hope you will use this book in two different ways. Sometimes, you may dip in and out of it for specific information about a particular drug. Suppose you are like Jill with the

bronchitis described above, you need to read about antibiotics in pregnancy. That bit of information could make your decision clearer. Anne could read about drugs for epilepsy. But the decision itself is only half the story. What I also want to explore, with women who want short, snappy summaries of the facts about a particular drug ('What about nystatin? Can I use that?'), are the underlying issues. Why did not Jill feel that she could take even an aspirin? Why was she so reluctant to ring her doctor? Why did she need the reassurance of a book like this after her doctor prescribed ampicillin? Was she reassured?

Unravelling these issues will help you make better decisions about *all* drugs in pregnancy and childbirth. That's what the first section of the book is for – to explore the issues behind the current epidemic of anxiety about drugs. You need to understand how we got into this situation, what the risks from drugs actually are, and when drug risks are at their greatest. It describes how limited our knowledge actually is concerning the effects of most drugs on pregnant women and their developing babies. And it looks at strategies that doctors and women themselves have developed to cope with the worry and responsibility of making decisions for mother and baby.

๛

Selecting which drugs to investigate

Listing hundreds of drugs and then writing 'Safety in pregnancy not established. Consult your doctor' (which is all I could write about most drugs available on prescription or over the counter) seemed to me a futile exercise. It also reinforces the false impression that your doctor might have the information which, in fact, isn't the case. This is not because he or she is negligent, but because the information does not exist. The drugs discussed in this book are the ones doctors talk to each other about in their professional journals and books. They are the ones that women have consistently been concerned about since I began working with pregnant women in the mid 1970s. If the drug you are looking for is not here, you might ask at your library, consult the British Medical Association's *Guide to Medicines and Drugs* (Dorling Kindersley) or the British National Formulary or talk to your doctor. You will probably discover that 'safety in pregnancy is not established', and then the chapters on coping with uncertainty might help (see Chapters 4 and 5).

Making good decisions takes time, effort, and the support of those around you. I hope that the information and discussion in this book will help you make the best choices possible, for yourself and your baby.

Author's note: There is a glossary at the back of the book which explains the special words and terms used in this book.

INTRODUCTION

✂ 1 ✂

What Lies Behind our Attitude to Drugs?

In the introduction I mentioned a woman who broke her ribs. The question was why the doctor didn't prescribe something for the pain. In one sense, the explanation is obvious. You need only one word: thalidomide. Even if the woman herself knew nothing of the tragedy that happened 35 years ago and even if her doctor did not consciously remind himself of the story, the shadow of thalidomide hung over the consulting room. It directly affected what the doctor did and how the woman felt about his decision. You cannot start to understand present attitudes towards drugs in pregnancy unless you start with thalidomide. It may reassure you to know in advance that I have concentrated on the folly of the drug manufacturers, rather than dwelling on the suffering of the victims.

✂
A Tragedy Unfolds

The first clue that something awful was happening came in 1961 with a short letter to a medical journal from an Australian obstetrician which said that he had recently delivered three babies, all of whom suffered from a condition he had not seen before. They had no arms but they did have fingers where their shoulders should be. As he had not seen this defect before and was staggered to see three cases so close together, he had interviewed the mothers. The only common thing he found was that they all had taken a widely-prescribed drug called thalidomide. Had anyone else noticed such a defect following thalidomide, he wondered?

The letters came back quickly reporting similar cases. In 1962, two German doctors published a study that 'blew the whistle' on thalidomide, though the argument as to whether or not the drug was the culprit raged for months. There was no argument about the result. Babies all over the world were being born without arms or legs and with other rare and distinctive abnormalities. In all, 10,000 deformed babies lived – many more were too severely damaged to survive. All their mothers had taken thalidomide in early pregnancy.

Thalidomide was developed in the 1950s by a German company, Chemie Grunenthal, who marketed it around the world. Its biggest selling point was the firm's claims that it was entirely safe and free of side-effects. Both claims are preposterous. To claim that it was entirely safe is to claim that there was no risk at all, but everything – every single choice – entails some risk. Risk is part of life. We now know that what we want from a drug is not to be risk free (that's impossible) but to have benefits which, on balance, make taking the drug worthwhile. Nothing can be 'entirely safe'.

To claim a drug has no side-effects is also astonishing. Every drug that is active enough to have a good effect will also have the potential of causing ill effects in some people. Again, it is a question of weighing the beneficial effect against how frequent or how serious the harmful effect might be.

Chemie Grunenthal didn't think that way. Indeed, they were so convinced by their own sales pitch that thalidomide was available in Germany until the end of the 1950s without prescription. Other countries were more cautious. One of the few positive aspects of this story was the scepticism of the American Federal Drug Administration when it was presented with Grunenthal's application to market the drug. One woman, Dr Frances Kelsey, was unconvinced; she asked for more tests to be done, thereby delaying the process for a few months. Those few months were long enough for the true danger of thalidomide to be discovered.

Frances Kelsey spared thousands of American babies from becoming Grunenthal's victims and their claim that the drug's 'safety' made it especially useful to pregnant women. Years later, when parents tried to claim compensation, they discovered that not only had the company done no tests on pregnant women to substantiate this claim, but that they had done no animal tests at all and only the crudest, most inadequate tests on its side-effects or safety in humans. They broke no laws and ignored no regulations because none existed at that time. Like all drug companies, Grunenthal were free to synthesize new drugs, to market them aggressively around the world if they wished, and to make grandiose claims as to their effectiveness. In this case, they claimed their product was unique in its safety.

Ironically, thalidomide was 'unique'. It was spectacularly damaging for human babies and human babies alone. A woman only had to take one pill between the twenty-seventh and thirty-third day of her pregnancy for it to cause nearly a 100 per cent chance of an instantly recognizable collection of deformities. Yet thalidomide caused almost no effects on most species of animals commonly used in drug tests (though, later, when they gave it to mice, they found changes which were in no way comparable to the devastating effects in humans, but which were worrying enough to signal the need for caution and further tests). The effects did not appear to be related to how much of the drug the mother took. And it was possible to determine precisely the time during which thalidomide could harm a baby. Mothers who took it outside those days by and large didn't have damaged babies. No drug developed before – or thankfully, since – even remotely resembles thalidomide in any of these characteristics.

Yet it took two years to notice that something was horribly wrong and two more to get the drug banned. Why? Because the laws governing the testing and sale of drugs were lax and based solely on the naïve view that drug companies would police themselves. They alone decided what drugs could or could not be sold. In retrospect, this absence of concern seems unbelievable but such was the tenor of the times. Everyone felt more relaxed about drugs. In Canada, half of the women who had affected children had not been prescribed the thalidomide they took. Though it was supposed to be available only on prescription, these women had accepted tablets from friends, drug salesmen or other casual sources.

Ever since, people have struggled to ensure that such a disaster does not happen again, and in the last 35 years much has changed. For one thing, the social climate differs. Diseases caused by medical treatment itself (called iaterogenic diseases) make big news stories – today we read of Opren patients suing drug companies and women forming pressure groups to seek compensation for damage by IUDs. It is hard to imagine those postwar days when it seemed as though pills could fix everything. Back then, breakthroughs like the discovery of penicillin meant that 1950s newspapers were full of 'miracle cures' and 'wonder drugs'.

Into this heady atmosphere dropped the shocking stories of children born without limbs. Things had to change, and they did. Governments enacted new laws regulating the manufacture, testing, and sale of drugs. They also insisted that drug companies monitor the effects of drugs on people. The new science of teratology – the study of abnormal development and causes of congenital malformations was born. The next chapter describes what teratologists have discovered in the last 35 years.

2

Teratology – The Study of Birth Defects

Teratology grew out of the searing experience of thalidomide, but from the moment it began, scientists were not the only ones interested in why fetal development sometimes went wrong. The media and the general public desperately wanted to know as well. Nobody could ever forget the photos of those thalidomide children.

From the beginning, the search had a high profile. Journalists lauded the energy and conviction of the scientists and, inadvertently, they also helped a misconception to grow. People believed that all the causes of birth defects were as clear-cut as thalidomide and that science knew already (or soon would know) what the causes might be. It followed, therefore, that birth defects could be prevented, and that doctors and drug companies were guilty of neglect when they did not do so. The facts do not support this.

The cause of birth defects

In 1992 just over 6,000 births with congenital malformations were recorded for England and Wales. To put this in proportion, about 88 per 10,000 – or less than one in every hundred – babies were born with serious abnormalities, and the figure has fallen from two in a hundred in 1982. Given this rate you would expect, on average, a hundred babies in every 11,300 deliveries to be abnormal – these are abnormalities which require immediate surgery or severely limit the child's quality of life; some are fatal. What goes wrong for these hundred babies?

What goes wrong for those 100 babies?

Seven children will have inherited a single abnormal gene present in the egg or sperm they received from their parents. Babies with sickle cell anaemia or cystic fibrosis fall into this category. Each has, in every cell in the body, one bad gene in a string of genes called a chromosome. It is like having one wrong bead on a necklace.

Six or so babies will have chromosomal abnormalities, in each cell they have one chromosome which is like one wrong necklace in a collection. The most common example of this is Down's Syndrome.

Six or seven children will have birth defects because of something that harmed them from the mother's environment. Of those six or seven, three on average may have been damaged by an infectious illness like rubella or cytomegalovirus, and less than one will have been harmed by a chronic illness, like diabetes, suffered by the mother. What is significant in the context of this book is that less than one per cent, or fewer than one in every hundred babies born with a serious abnormality, can be directly linked to a prescription or over-the-counter drug. Even though recent studies from a number of countries have shown that more than 80 per cent of women take one or more drugs during pregnancy. That one child could well be damaged by drugs the mother *had* to take for her own health, or something she took inadvertently before she knew of the pregnancy.

The rest will have defects that have less well defined causes. 20 children will have disorders developed in the uterus because they inherited a tendency towards the condition and something in the fetal environment triggered off this tendency. One example might be central nervous system disorders like spina bifida. Another might be the Fetal Alcohol Syndrome (see page 134), a distinctive cluster of abnormalities found in some babies born to alcoholics.

And, finally, as many as 60 per cent will have serious abnormalities for which no indentifiable cause can be found.

ﭘ

A note about minor abnormalities

Most of this book focuses on major anomalies – the ones that threaten a baby's life, health or quality of life. Depending on how you classify 'minor', between seven and ten babies in every hundred have one or more characteristics not found in the other 90 or so babies. These minor abnormalities can either be ignored or easily corrected, and the possibilities are huge – an extra finger, or a birth mark, or a hip joint that is too loose.

Though called 'minor', these can and do cause parents worry and pain. They vary in their feelings about such problems: some take them in their stride; others find it hard to come to terms with a problem that experts regard as temporary and correctable. They deserve help and support just as parents of more damaged babies do. Nevertheless, most study and effort is devoted to major abnormalities because the consequences are more devastating for the baby and the family.

ﭘ

Living with uncertainty

We do not know what causes most birth defects. Even after 35 years of research, we can identify the specific cause in only a tiny number of abnormal births, and of those, drugs in general do not appear to be a major factor. Many people quickly point out that what went wrong in the unexplained abnormal births could well have been caused by environmental factors, too. That may be. Or drugs could act as potentiators, a sort of trigger, in the 60 per cent of cases where there is no understood cause.

There is no room for complacency nor must we relax our guard lest anything as awful as the thalidomide disaster occur again. But most experts who review the field of teratology conclude with a reassuring message. Drs Heinonen, Kline and Shapiro declared, after an exhaustive review of 50,000 mother-baby pairs between 1959 and 1965, when prescription drug use rates were much higher than they are now. 'No commonly used drugs were identified whose potency as teratogens could be regarded as even remotely comparable to thalidomide ...' and, after reviewing the literature on birth defects concluded, 'Drugs in general are not an important factor in congenital malformation in general.'

Unlike the reassuring claims made by drug manufacturers in the fifties, such statements are now based on research done all over the world. Now, if he had the time or inclination, your doctor could read dozens of new research journals which publish papers describing thousands of experiments costing millions of pounds. What is intriguing is that doctors are not reassured, and neither are parents. To the extent that reassurance might lull them into dangerous complacency, I am grateful for that. But to what extent does their refusal to accept this conclusion lead to bad decisions and too much worrying? One study shows that both do happen.

In 1985, a clinic in Toronto, Canada, was set up to counsel women who had been exposed to drugs, chemicals or radiation in the first third of pregnancy. In 1989, the authors published a study in which they asked 80 women who came to their clinic about what they felt about the risks from these three dangers. How likely did they think it was that their baby was damaged? All the women assessed the risk of birth defects to the population in general fairly accurately (about 5 per cent), yet they assigned themselves 'substantial teratogenic risk in the range assigned to that of thalidomide'. Even after counselling, when women were told that the drug or chemical was *not* thought to be deforming, they still thought they ran risks of around 14 per cent, over three times that of the general population. Women who took drugs known to be teratogenic but necessary for their own health thought they had a 36 per cent risk of having a damaged child (i.e. 1 in 3). This is wildly inaccurate. Epileptic women, for example, must take drugs that are among the most teratogenic regularly prescribed to patients, yet 94 in every 100 will have a perfectly normal child.

This level of anxiety is disturbing on two grounds. Firstly, many women asked for and received terminations, based on their distorted impressions about risk. And secondly, most were sent to the specialist clinic by their family doctors, who had an equally inaccurate view of what was and was not dangerous and how risky a substance might be. The authors met 'many instances in which physicians advised women to abort after exposure to drugs not known to be risky'. There is a high price to pray for false perceptions.

ॐ

The origins of our distorted views

Why have we got it so wrong? Scientists and clinicians continue to place a great deal of attention on drugs and environmental influences. People get the idea that both must be very risky indeed to warrant all this effort. That's not quite accurate. It is not that these factors are the most dangerous or important, it is that they may be preventable. Pinpoint the cause and you can prevent the damage – something you cannot do for most abnormalities where no cause is known. This is effort well spent if even a tiny number of babies are spared, and recent research which shows that folate plays an important role in reducing the risk of spina bifida is a good example of what can be done.

One reason; however, why amongst all the environmental factors, drugs, in particular, receive so much attention is that one can choose whether or not to take a drug, smoke a cigarette or drink a glass of wine. Since there is a choice (in theory at least, if not always in practice), money and energy have been poured into influencing people's actions. It has not poured into educating people about the other causes of birth defects, because we do not know what they might be.

Public education campaigns give women a false picture of how much control and therefore responsibility they must bear for the eventual outcome of the pregnancy. When a baby is born with a defect, everyone searches for a cause. I remember a sad, withdrawn woman I saw on a television documentary describing the operation to reshape her eleven-week-old baby's deformed heart. She never spoke, never looked at the camera and rarely glanced at her husband. Only once in the hour-long programme did we hear her voice; a voice-over recording said, 'I keep thinking it was something I took ... some pill ... for a headache or something ...' and her voice trailed off into sad silence.

I wished I could have comforted her, listened to her express how guilty she feels, then helped her understand that she was not to blame. She did nothing to cause it and overlooked nothing that could have prevented it. I wished I could help her turn from blaming herself to giving help and support to her partner and receiving his in return. Together, they could help their baby in this terrible time, but she was locked in misery.

Parents need realistic ideas about what the dangers might be and when those dangers are greatest. Knowing this will not make the worry go away because no book, no study, no support group or explanation will ever make anxiety disappear completely. Women have always worried about the health of their babies and the worry doesn't stop with birth. Women – parents – do whatever they can to ensure that the baby is well. They can do this more effectively if they know something about how drugs might change the normal growth and development of their baby. That is what the next chapter is about. But they also need to remember how small a part drug decisions play in the overall wellbeing of their babies.

3

Drugs and Your Changing Baby

Each new life starts as one egg and one sperm; after nine months, a newborn baby made up of billions and billions of cells squeezes its way into the world. Almost always, the wet wide-eyed new baby is evidence that a process so complex it is mind-boggling has once again worked well.

When it does not, one of two things has happened. Either something was wrong with the genetic code that the baby received from the egg and sperm – about 35 per cent of abnormalities are genetic in origin. Or something harmed the baby during his or her development – 65 per cent of abnormalities fall into this category. As Chapter 2 points out, most abnormalities will not be attributable to any one agent so we cannot say *what* harmed them. We have a better chance of saying *when* the harm took place. This information is useful to you should you need to judge the risk if you take a drug inadvertently or if you need to weigh up risk and benefit of a future drug decision. The risk to your baby will vary depending on what stage of development he or she has reached.

Until about Day 15 (that's four weeks after the first day of your last period) each individual cell is 'multipotential'. That means any one cell could go on to develop into a variety of different forms and functions. Damage at this stage of development either results in repair by other cells or a miscarriage because of death of the whole embryo. There is more about particular dangers in Chapter 6 on preconception.

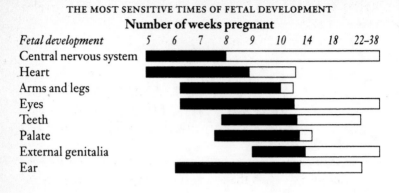

THE MOST SENSITIVE TIMES OF FETAL DEVELOPMENT
Number of weeks pregnant

■ high sensitivity   □ lower sensitivity

The duration of pregnancy is taken from the first day of the last period.

The next stage of any baby's development takes place largely between Day 15 and Day 56, though we must be careful not to stick too rigidly to these dates. This period starts about the time that your period was due and lasts for the next two to two and a half months. The first third of your pregnancy, while cells are becoming organs, is the time when babies are probably most sensitive to harm from teratogens. This is the time to be most wary of dangers like abdominal X-rays, heavy drinking, certain viruses, and some maternal illnesses (see page 20). And drugs. That does not mean that you should be *unwary* at other times, but that the baby's organs are changing and developing more rapidly than at any other time. Damage then will mean structural defects in the developing baby. The earlier in this period the damage occurs, the more serious the effect is likely to be.

By Day 56 or so (or twelve weeks in a baby's life and 14 weeks of pregnancy), most organs are fully formed, except a baby's teeth, genitals and brain; these remain vulnerable to structural damage. Brain cells in particular continue to multiply and differentiate until the baby is a toddler. Only at about 18 months do children have a central nervous system similar to an adult's. Drugs that are known to effect these organs continue to be teratogenic beyond the first twelve weeks.

Once organs are formed, drugs have effects that are much more similar to those found in adults.

- *They may change how the baby behaves* – For example, if the mother takes diazepam (valium) for a few weeks before birth, the baby will be born sleepy, unwilling to suck and unable to keep warm.
- *They may change how well a baby grows* – For example, cigarettes interfere with the amount of oxygen available, so the baby grows less well and is smaller than it would be otherwise.
- *They may reach the baby in doses that are fine for a grown woman but far too large for a baby* – Women taking heart medications need to monitor the baby's heart, too, in case it receives too much medication.
- *They give the baby harmful side-effects* – Streptomycin, a drug used to treat tuberculosis, is known to damage hearing if it is used for a long time; for this reason, it is recommended that it never be given to pregnant women.

There are other factors about taking a particular drug that influence the risk to the baby besides the stage of development reached; how often a woman takes the drug, how much she takes, and what other drug she is also taking all influence the effect on the baby. Because there are so many variables, it is very difficult to be sure, even if the drug is known to be risky, what the risks might be. The next two chapters consider how doctors and mothers cope with this and other uncertainties about drugs in pregnancy.

⁊ 4 ⁊

Coping With Uncertainty –
The Doctors' Dilemma

Teratologists do not under-
stand much about how most drugs affect developing babies,
and they are unlikely ever to know much about many. Doctors,
and women themselves, have evolved strategies for coping
with this uncertainty. This chapter looks at why this is so and
the way many doctors decide about drugs in pregnancy. The
next chapter deals with how women do this.

Two thirds of all the drugs currently available on prescription have no background data whatsoever about their effect on
pregnant women and their babies, and for the other third,
most of the information is vague and unhelpful. If a drug says
'Not recommended for pregnant women' on the packet, it
probably means that no real evidence exists one way or the
other. The same applies to the phrase 'contraindicated in
pregnancy' without any citation of adverse effects or studies
done to assess risk. They are phrases used by pharmaceutical
companies to serve the company rather than to offer guidance
to the doctor, and to cover their backs in case of law suits.

Drug companies are not taking steps to rectify this situation. Their duty is to test and study any new drug that is
coming on the market, and they do not test new drugs on
pregnant women. Much information that is available is based
on studies in animals. The reasons for not testing new drugs
on pregnant women are to some extent practical and ethical
and to a greater extent, financial. To discover any links
between drug x and birth defect y, a drug company would have

to study a large number of women. A research team at Guy's Hospital in London estimated that if a drug doubled the incidence of a specific serious malformation from one baby in 1000 births to two babies in every 1000 (which is quite a big effect), they would have to study 23,000 women who had been exposed to the drug, before they could prove this – before they could know that the effect happened more often than they would expect it to by chance. Finding sufficient numbers of women willing to take the drug would be a formidable task given the present climate of opinion, and the cost of trying would be prohibitive. As a result no newly developed drugs are being tested on pregnant women, and doctors cope with this by not prescribing them to pregnant patients.

ᘐ

Spotting Trouble

That leaves the thousands and thousands of drugs currently available on prescription, and the tens of thousands available without prescriptions, all with no clear guidelines. Some effort is going into spotting any that might cause problems. Doctors are asked to fill in a form reporting any adverse drug effects their patients might have suffered. One-off anomalies are often reported in the medical literature (along the lines of 'I had a patient who took drug X and her baby had such and such wrong with it …'). From time to time, large scale surveys are undertaken, such as the ones done in the early 1980s concerning the antinausea drug, Debendox (see page 84).

One way doctors cope with having insufficient knowledge is to prescribe drugs with a long track record. They reason that if a particular drug has been used for a long time by many women, chances are good that doctors would have noticed any problems.

That does not mean that commonly used drugs are safe, that we can ever prove them to be safe, or that doctors would necessarily spot an effect if one were present. One would only show up if the resulting defect was:

17

- *quite specific* – It might be possible to discover that something causes a very particular problem – say, a hand defect – though one must remember that it took months to notice the extreme consequences of thalidomide. And it is exceedingly difficult to devise tests for subtle effects like causing slower growth or a shorter attention span.
- *fairly frequent* – You would need to study hundreds of thousands of cases to spot something that happened in only a few of them. One doctor would never treat enough women to notice.
- *clearly identified as a problem* – All of us are 'abnormal' in so far as we are different from each other – we have bodies and ways of behaving that are unique to us. We just get on with living with our less-than-perfect selves. We will never know if our quirks are 'significant' or what might have caused them.

Unless a drug causes distinct harm in a pretty large proportion of babies the chances of spotting it are slim. But it does happen. An example is the anti-acne drug, isotretinoin, prescribed to teenagers. Some then went on to become pregnant, with disastrous results. A 1984 report of 34 pregnancies, describes only 15 live-born children of whom 10 were severely handicapped. The drug and other retinoids such as acitretin, are now given more cautiously, and always with contraception. Individual vigilance is probably the best way we have of identifying drugs that could be dangerous to a developing baby, and it is the way most of the drugs now known to be dangerous have been spotted.

꒰

Avoiding known risks

It would be wrong to suppose doctors are always uncertain. Medical literature regularly publishes lists of drugs known to be teratogenic. These drugs will not hurt every baby or even the majority of babies who are exposed to them, but the risks have been measured and found to be well above the risk levels present if the drug is *not* taken. Many of the drugs in this list are described in more detail in later chapters.

Experts do not all agree what is and is not teratogenic but here is a list published in the report of a 1988 conference of world experts on birth defects. It is divided into three sections. One section lists substances known to damage babies. They include 16 drugs or chemicals (see list over).

This list is *not* the definitive list but it is fairly representative of many such lists (to this list could be added other anti-convulsant drugs for epilepsy such as carbamazepine and phenobarbitol, because of the evidence of risk of fetal damage; as could sintrom, another drug for clotting disorders; clorniphene, an ovulation stimulating drug; high doses of vitamin A; and inhibitors which are drugs for hypertension). Your doctor will probably have seen similar lists and would only prescribe a drug from this list if there was no alternative, and because the risks were outweighed by the benefits.

ॐ

Deciding when the risks are not well known

The British National Formulary advises 'drugs should only be prescribed during pregnancy if the expected benefit to the mother is thought to be greater than the risk to the fetus, and all drugs should be avoided if possible during the first trimester'. And so the most common way doctors cope with not knowing whether a drug is safe enough is by being extremely reluctant to prescribe *anything* to pregnant women. They do this both because they are afraid of being wrong, and because they are afraid of being sued.

A British child has the right to take his or her mother's doctor to court for damage done *in utero* or at birth until he or she is 21. Parents, too, can sue. In North America, the rush to law has become a stampede in recent years. In 1985, 60 per cent of American obstetricians has been sued at least once. Any American doctor you come across is likely to have several

Drug/Chemical	Condition Treated
Aminopterin	cancer
Androgenic hormones (eg testosterone)	cancer
Busulfan (busulphan)	cancer
Chlorobiphenyls	(toxic chemicals)
Cyclosphosphamide	cancer
Diethylstilbestrol	cancer
Heroin/methodone	
Iodide	hyperthyroidism
Isotretinoin	acne/psoriasis
Lithium carbonate	manic-depression
Phenytoin	epilepsy
Propylthiouracil	hyperthyroidism
Tetracycline	infection/acne
Trimethadione	epilepsy
Valproic Acid	epilepsy
Warfarin	clotting disorders

Two heavy metals:
lead   mercury
And radiation, specifically cancer therapy, where the dose to fetus is large.

The list also includes seven infectious diseases that are known to harm a developing baby. They are:

rubella
syphilis
toxoplasmosis
cytomegalovirus
herpes simplex virus
varicella
Venezuelan equine encephalitis virus

And seven conditions or actions present in the mother regarded as dangerous:

alcoholism
insuline-dependent diabetes*
maternal phenylketonuria (PKU)*
Myasthenia gravis*
myotonic dystrophy*
smoking
systematic lupus erythmatosus*

* These are all chronic illnesses. If you have no idea what they are, you are not a sufferer and you have nothing to worry about! (Author's note)
    Source: Transplacental Effects on Fetal Health ed. Scarpelli and Migaki (Liss) 1988, p. 178.

lawsuits in progress at any one time. The same is not yet true in Britain. British people react with incredulity to cases like Grodin *vs* Grodin, a suit brought by a child against his own mother for taking the drug tetracycline (an antibiotic) in pregnancy – the drug caused the child's teeth to be discoloured. But British doctors do *talk* about being sued, many worry about it and a few actually are. Most will go to some lengths to avoid the possibility.

This has changed obstetrics in the last decades. It has meant more tests and interventions, and fewer drugs. Some women have scan after scan, 'just in case', they are hospitalized 'just in case', they are induced 'just in case' ... It explains why there are so many false positives when doctors look for intrauterine growth retardation and why the manufacturers of electronic fetal monitoring were so successful in marketing their machines. When a senior doctor advises his junior, his words are so often, 'Well, we better have a look at it just in case ...' The opposite attitude holds for drugs. Not more, less. As one American doctor told me, 'You can be sued more easily for what you do prescribe than what you don't.'

Naturally, that is not the only reason for caution. Doctors do not want to be wrong. They read journals, attend seminars, listen to colleagues and assemble as much information as they can before making decisions. But that is not always enough. Prescribing for pregnant women means that doctors must make decisions in the face of uncertainty. They know that colleagues in the past have made mistakes and that they are not immune. This can lead to what one observer called 'pharmacological nihilism' – denying treatment to women who need it and who would benefit from drugs. However, some doctors do prescribe or medical literature would not include regular articles warning them not to do so. One doctor that did concluded, 'When treatment is necessary, it should be instituted, as untreated maternal illness may be harmful to the developing fetus.'

◌

Whose risk and whose benefit?

One way doctors seek to simplify these complicated decisions is to give unequal weight to the needs of the mother and baby. In its most extreme form this can lead doctors to treat women merely as vessels carrying a baby. The results of such an attitude can be very extreme as the legal cases cited on page 170 show. On a more mundane level, they can make decisions like the one described in the first chapter of this book – denying a woman with broken ribs any pain relief because she was four months pregnant. Maura (a name I have given her) said, 'When I was four months pregnant, I broke two ribs. The doctor refused to give me anything for the pain and I was in agony for months. It hurt every single time I breathed.'

In one sense, the doctor's decision made sense. Even though Maura's growing baby had already passed the most vulnerable time (the first twelve weeks of life) it was still at risk. The baby's brain was still developing and all organ systems were continuing to mature and grow. The doctor will be keen to prevent any teratogen from reaching the baby, and Maura, of course, will be even keener to keep harm at bay.

Any pain killer the doctor might prescribe carries some risk that it is teratogenic. One study of 50,000 women showed that taking codeine during pregnancy was associated with a very small increase in the number of children born with lung malformations. Did the codeine cause this? We do not know, it could equally have been the result of whatever illness led the woman to take the drug in the first place. In this case, Maura was 16 weeks pregnant and her baby's lungs were probably fully formed. The British Medical Association's *Guide to Medicines and Drugs* states that codeine has 'no evidence of risk' for the baby, and there are other painkillers which have similar evidence.

Maura's doctor looked at the choices and concluded, 'I can't tell you it's safe, so I won't prescribe anything.' He decided that weighing up the risk – however tiny – to the baby and the benefit of relief from pain – however great – for the mother, justified doing nothing. He could be right. But he could have looked at the consequences too narrowly. By doing so, he treated Maura not as a person in her own right, but as the container for her growing baby.

Maura is not, actually, an unfeeling suitcase – she is a person with needs and reactions that deserve recognition. To truly balance out the risks and benefits of denying her pain relief, you must also consider the consequence of being in pain for several months. What might they be?

- *More stress* – Pain is disruptive, tiring and very stressful. Maura probably produced large quantities of stress hormones – chemicals like epinepherine and norepinepherine – which have a direct effect on the uterine muscle, and may be the reason why women experiencing high levels of stress have an increased risk of premature labour.

   Stress may also be teratogenic though evidence is somewhat equivocal in humans. Its effects on animals are much clearer: pregnant mice who were artificially stressed gained less weight because they ate and drank less. Their offspring were more vulnerable to stress themselves and showed abnormal sexual development because their hormone levels were below normal. In sorting out the causes of the offspring's abnormal behaviour, one scientist noted, 'Stress alters behaviour in many ways that mimic drug exposure *per se*.' Mice are not the same as people, but we do produce chemicals in response to stress. They have an effect and evidence suggests they also affect a developing baby. So by denying Maura pain relief because of the tiny risk, the doctor did not keep risk at bay, he merely changed it to that caused by stress.

- *Negative feelings* – Even if sustained pain caused no physical changes in Maura's developing baby, it certainly changed how she felt about the pregnancy and about her baby. It is normal to resent the discomforts and limitations that pregnancy causes – we all feel that sometimes. But as the months pass, most of us feel a growing attachment to the coming baby that keeps the resentment in perspective. Maura had more than most women to feel angry about and although she never expressed that feeling in any way except words, not all women can show such restraint.

An American psychiatrist who has studied prenatal physical abuse reports that 8 per cent of pregnant women and 9 per cent of their partners describe feeling the urge to retaliate against the baby by physically assaulting it. Some actually do though this is probably rare. According to this author, his findings are greeted with incredulity and denial in the same way that many reacted to early reports of child abuse.

So it is not so straightforward a matter to weigh up risk and benefit after all – especially when the risk is unknown and is borne by one person and the benefit by the other! Clearly, too, it is not a decision that involves only the doctor. Maura, too, needs to be in on it – and in this case, she was not. Both of them need to take time to consider the risks and benefits in as wide a way as possible.

This message will recur throughout this book. How important it is to look at the issues as widely as possible. How important it is to take time to consider. How impossible it is to ever know if you have made the *right* decision. These matters are difficult and it is not only doctors who find them so. The next chapter looks at ways that women cope with very similar dilemmas. Many use the same strategies described for doctors but because the issues are different, they have also devised some of their own.

5

Estimating Risk and Benefit – The Mother's Dilemma

A former American president, Harry Truman, had a sign on his desk saying 'the buck stops here.' That's how it is for pregnant women and drug decisions. For the general public, there are academic questions about relative risks, or political questions about the role of drug companies or the responsibilities of government. For doctors, drug decisions may touch feelings of professional competence, fears about litigation or philosophical questions about whether or not a woman is a vessel for her baby. But for the woman herself, these questions touch her own life and her own baby. Everyone makes decisions about drugs on grounds other than the purely rational as we have already seen, but how the mother feels matters just as much as what she knows.

How women feel about drug decisions varies widely but most women will readily admit that they feel fiercely protective towards their unborn child. They will do all they can to safeguard their precious, utterly dependent, and as yet unknown, person. Most feel all sorts of conflicts about whose needs to put first.

For most drugs, it seems as though the woman gets all the benefit and the baby carries all the risk. But that's not the whole picture – a baby can also benefit from living inside a mother who is as well as she can be, even if sometimes a drug is needed to help her be so. But it does not feel that way, just as it does not always feel as though two people's needs deserve to be considered. Despite all the feminist rhetoric, most women still believe they should subjugate their own needs to those of others, a belief that is magnified a hundredfold once they become pregnant. If a woman wavers from this view, her family and friends will soon remind her that she must 'Think of the Baby'. I remember one antenatal teacher who, when I asked her how she would answer a query from a pregnant woman as to whether or not she should take aspirin for a headache, sharply shot back, 'I'd tell her she was only doing it for selfish reasons.' When told that there was no evidence that occasional aspirins are harmful (see page 109), she did not alter this view. Protectiveness and altruism make choices even harder.

So, too, does a powerful sense of responsibility. In time, most parents do grow used to making choices on behalf of their children but first time parents in particular often find the burden of responsibility very heavy. It is not surprising, then, that they focus more earnestly on dangers than benefits and it would be wrong to suggest they do not. But it will help in deciding matters if they do not lose track of the benefits of drugs too.

༜

The benefits of drugs

Newspapers are less likely to print stories that detail the *value* or drugs for pregnant women than their dangers. Because of prescribed drugs women have conceived who would not have done so; they have carried a pregnancy through when they would otherwise have lost the baby; and they kept harm at bay for themselves and their babies. Our daily lives too are healthier, longer and more comfortable because of drugs. Antimalarial pills gave me protection when I worked in Africa; anti-asthma medication allows my husband to live a normal life; my son was kept pain-free after an operation, my daughter recovered from pneumonia; and my youngest did not spend his toddlerhood with bad hearing from repeated ear infections. You, too, must be familiar with similar benefits.

We all know, however, that this is only half of the story and simply to point to the good drugs do could appear naïve or complacent. No one who has delved into the past catastrophes and tragedies connected with drugs can only see the rosy side. I know that when it comes to how drugs are researched, manufactured, marketed and prescribed much could be improved.

I know drugs cause side-effects. One estimate reckons that a new drug coming on the market could be expected to cause different side-effects in 40 per cent of the people who take it. That is why we need the best information available to help us decide whether or not to take it. After all, if a drug cured cancer and had the unfortunate side-effect of causing baldness, it would be hailed as a miracle. If, on the other hand, it cured baldness and had the unfortunate side-effect of causing cancer in even a small number of people, no responsible physician would prescribe it and no thinking patient would accept it if he did. But the problem with most drugs is they fall well short of either extreme.

Despite all these reservations, drugs in general are more beneficial than harmful as anyone who has spent time in Third World countries, where few are available and the need overwhelming, would testify. Decisions about each particular drug, however, can still be a closely argued point, and few cases are more problematic than those involving decisions when you are pregnant.

࿎

Making hard choices even harder

Over the years, I have watched parents struggling to decide what to do about many things including drugs in pregnancy. I've noticed three things that seem to make this even harder: understanding and using statistics; falling for fallacies about risk; and striving for the impossible, for example, a risk-free pregnancy. It may help you to look at these three points before you begin making decisions based on the information in the chapters ahead.

Statistics – bane and boon

Good academic studies finish with numbers – 'twice the risk of this' or 'a significant measure of that'. This is satisfying for the research team and for the reader – we may be one step closer to Truth. There is no doubt that having figures makes deciding easier in many ways and the language we use even implies this when we talk of 'weighing up' risk and benefit. In fact, few of us make up our minds like that. Why not?

Statistics may not be helpful because many other factors besides just the statistics are involved in decisions – most of them cannot be quantified. Take the example of a woman, aged 34, who has to decide whether or not to have an amniocentesis to discover if the baby she is carrying has Down's syndrome. She is told that, on average, 1.23 women per 1000 in the age group 30–34 years old have a Down's baby. Amniocentesis, however, results in miscarriage for five women in every 1000 tested. Do the statistics make her choice any easier? Will they make the decision?

The chances are that you would be unlikely to reject amniocentesis purely because you are five times more likely to lose the baby by miscarriage than to have a Down's baby. Instead you think about how you feel about having a Down's baby … how long you tried to get pregnant … how your partner feels … how you view abortion – all these values probably carry more weight than the relative risk values.

Also, statistics may not be helpful because statistics for one person are not necessarily applicable to another. Knowing that, on average, five women per thousand have a baby with a certain abnormality if they take drug x will not tell you what the risk is for you. Each person is unique and the way a drug acts on each of us is unique. How likely it is for you will depend on your genetic make-up, your baby's genetic make-up, your baby's stage of development, how much of the drug you take, how long you take it and so on. These factors make it hard to know if the result found in a large group applies to you, though the larger the group and the more carefully the study designers tried to untangle them, the more likely it is to be relevant for you.

Statistics may not be helpful because they cannot predict the future. The best study in the world will not say what will happen to you for sure, though it can mean closer and closer guesses. The most we can look for is a sort of bookmaker's guide to risk.

They may not be helpful because they are prone to misleading the reader as well as informing. Since we do not usually think in statistical terms, it is hard to get the messages they bring straight. It may help to remember:

- Statistics usually describe all-or-nothing events. If they happen, it is 100 per cent; if they do not, it is zero. A 20 per cent increase in risk does not mean a 20 per cent increase in effect.

- Statistics lend themselves to the 'half empty/half full syndrome' because they can be made to appear either good or bad depending on the emphasis. For example, to say a drug doubles the chances that your baby could be damaged sounds grim news. Or you might say that if 1000 women all took the drug, we would expect 998 to have a healthy baby and two babies to have a particular deformity; if none took the drug, we could expect 999 babies to not have the defect and one to have it. They mean the same but the second example sounds more reassuring – except, of course, if yours is that one baby.

- Statistics can only draw conclusions about things you can quantify – if you can count it, statisticians are interested. They go for well defined, uncomplicated situations like the one that kept a friend of mine busy for years – measuring the internal temperature of carnation buds. She became very accurate at assessing the causes of one effect or another on her flowers. On the other hand human beings, thank heavens, are rather more complicated than carnations. Our fears, religious beliefs, experiences in childhood and count- less other factors, influence what we do and how things affect us, but they are very hard to turn into numbers.

When no statistics exist

It is all very well to be reminded that numbers and statistics and known risk values are not sufficient to make decisions ... but they are still very useful! *Not* having any idea of what the risk might be is worse than no help at all – it prevents you from making up your mind. Unfortunately, it is more often the case that we know too few statistics than that we are troubled by too many when it comes to drugs in pregnancy.

Even if the packet insert accompanying a drug mentions specific risks, you get little idea of the size of that risk. How many babies are affected? When are the most vulnerable times? It may not say. So what do you do? You could consult books like this to see what evidence there is, you could talk to the hospital pharmacist or ask your doctor. You could fall back on decision-making strategies you have used in the past. Though these strategies are often based on fallacies, they do have the advantage of allowing people to act, rather than leaving them paralysed with doubt. Remember, decisions do have to be made and if you don't make them, someone else will.

The 'you've got to try' fallacy

Many people believe (though few would say so) that, given two options, doing nothing is irresponsible but doing something – even though it may be risky – proves that you've done your best. You've tried.

It is on exactly this basis that victims of the drug, DES (diethylstilbestrol), now forgive their mothers who took it when they were pregnant. In 1937, the first synthetic hormone was made in a laboratory – diethylstilbestrol – and with it, doctors could directly influence the female reproductive cycle. Doctors began prescribing it in 1945 for women who had experienced a miscarriage in a previous pregnancy because, after the War, everyone was desperate to start a family and they wanted to do something to help when the first attempt failed. Perhaps, they reasoned, a hormone would help, so they tried and noticed that few women had a second miscarriage. No trials were done to show DES had anything to do with this.

Then in 1953, a double-blind control trial showed that DES was no better than a placebo at preventing miscarriage; indeed, women given the drug did worse than those without. But the trial had little clinical impact. Between 1959 and 1965, 2.3 million American women were prescribed DES 'to prevent miscarriage'. Four thousand women in Great Britain took DES (called stilboestrol in the UK).

In 1970, disturbing reports of very young women with clear-cell carcinoma of the cervix began to appear. It turns out that one woman in 1000 exposed to DES *in utero* develops a rare form of cancer of the vagina and cervix. DES is the only known chemical that crosses the placenta and causes cancer in the offspring. More recently (1995) there have been reports of adenocarcinoma of the vagina in older DES exposed women. Many DES daughters – some reports say as many as 90 per cent – have abnormalities of the reproductive organs that make conception difficult, contraception more problematic, increase rates of miscarriage and cause various other difficulties.

DES sons are also affected. They have many more genital abnormalities; many have a low sperm count and they are more likely to have undescended or undeveloped testicles. We know less about the full effect in DES sons because the publicity is biased towards the daughters and cancers typically develop later in men.

I tell the DES story here to show how powerful the 'You've got to try' fallacy can be. One doctor, looking back at the DES experience, explained, 'Women who have lost babies and those desperate to conceive a child, are groups from whom it is difficult to withhold a drug that the physician thinks might be helpful. This possibility can lead clinical investigators who are responsive to their patients, to overlook the absence of proper trials.' Apparently, this argument is accepted by their patients because not one has filed a suit against her own gynaecologist, though many hundreds of suits have been filed against the drug companies manufacturing the drug. (Cynics would say this is just because the companies have more money but surely women could sue both?)

A DES daughter, writing after her hysterectomy, says, 'Mom has always felt so terrible about taking this pill that caused me cancer – even though she knew that she had taken it only because she had wanted to have me so badly.' She bore no grudge because she understood that, for her mother, it seemed right to do something rather than nothing – even if the risks of acting turned out to be greater.

The 'if I do nothing it's not my fault' fallacy

Sometimes, people find the consequences that flow from doing something are much more onerous to bear than the ones that come from *not* doing something. This way it's 'Nature's Way'.

That is the only possible explanation for parents who refuse to allow their newborn baby to be vaccinated against whooping cough. The chance that the vaccine will damage the baby is miniscule – about one in 300,000 babies – while the chances of the baby contracting the disease are very real. Indeed, every year of the several hundred thousand babies born in the UK (793,000 in 1991), between four and seven will die from whooping cough; dozens will be permanently damaged and hundreds will suffer weeks or months of coughing. Yet parents refuse the injection. One explained to me that if she agreed and the baby was damaged, she would never forgive herself but if her baby caught the illness, well, that was fate, wasn't it?

The 'doing nothing has no risks' fallacy

The more you feel uneasy about the risks, the more you might opt for this belief, and because drugs make pregnant women uneasy they impose an absolute ban on them. This may actually increase the risks to the baby. For example, if a woman has a fever, the most helpful thing for her baby is to reduce the fever as soon as possible. Many women will not do this because they are afraid of the side-effects of drugs in general, and aspirin or paracetamol in particular. Neither drug is associated with miscarriage but fever is (see page 111). Some illnesses in pregnancy can potentially harm the baby and need to be treated (see Chapters 8 and 9). In these cases *something* lessens the risk.

The 'daily life risks don't count' fallacy

Another strategy people use is to consider only some risks as important and disregard others. Consider the woman whose story comes up in the chapter on alcohol. She had two drinks in early pregnancy, before she knew she was pregnant, and then worried herself sick about the risks to her baby for the next nine months. At the same time, she used the M1 twice a week to get to and from work. The chances of the two drinks harming the baby were, depending on the study you read, either very small indeed or non-existent. The chances that she might be in a car crash were many times greater, yet she never considered them.

Being risk free: the most tempting fantasy of all

By living, we put ourselves and our babies at risk – we have no other option. Of course, we have a responsibility to mini-mize the dangers before we act. I look both ways before I cross the street, but I do cross streets. And because we are responsible for our children, we have to think hard about risk before making decisions for them. But I do choose some things that involve risk. I hold their hand tightly when they are two; explain how to cross when they turn five; teach them to cross when they are seven; and then cross my fingers and watch them do it alone when they are about eight. But I let them do it. I have no choice and I do not want their lives or mine blighted by a futile effort to try and guarantee their safety.

The same holds true in pregnancy. You will have to make decisions that will by necessity involve risk. You will find information in the chapters ahead to help you make up your mind about what drugs to take or avoid in pregnancy. The more you know about a drug, the better your decision will be. The more you know about yourself, the more likely your decision will be right for you. The more you evaluate whatever you decide – not to blame yourself but to understand how and why you make that choice – the more likely you will consider all the risks and benefits for you and your baby the next time.

PRECONCEPTION AND EARLY PREGNANCY

Drugs Before Pregnancy

Preconception* –
three different approaches

For a few women, the time between making up their mind to try for a baby and the moment when the pregnancy test is positive can be very busy. They plan their preconception, drop some old habits, learn a bit about what is good for growing babies and generally get ready for the adventure ahead.

It is certainly a time that fills some parents with energy and enthusiasm. One said:

> I like to be organized about things. You should have seen me when Bruce and I got married – my Mum and I were at it for months. I think it's crazy that people do more research before buying a washing machine than about having a baby. Three months ago, I didn't know what preconception was, now I've got books from the library, and checklists for both of us, and even daily vitamin pills.

---

* By 'preconception' parents usually mean the time between stopping contraception and a positive pregnancy test. It ends when the baby has been developing for as few as three weeks. Doctors usually consider that it extends to the first antenatal visit when the mother is officially registered as pregnant. By then, her baby may have been growing for 10 to 12 weeks. For this chapter, the parents definition seems most useful – 'preconception' stops when you are pretty sure you are pregnant.

Other couples may be just as keen to start a pregnancy but do not take this approach. They just stop contraception and see what happens.

> I've been pretty health conscious for the past few years. Pete and I think about what we eat, and neither of us smokes or drinks much anyway. I figure that millions of women in the world who are less healthy than I am have babies, so my chances are at least as good as theirs. I'm not perfect so why should I expect the baby to be?

Of course, some parents have no choice because they discover that a baby is on the way. Somewhere between twenty and forty babies in every hundred are unplanned and these mothers and fathers can only look back and wonder if anything they did inadvertently will have an effect on their developing baby.

When it comes to the kind of pregnancy you will experience or the health of the baby, does in matter if you are someone who plans ahead, the sort who waits to see, or the frankly surprised? A new medical field called Preconceptual Care is starting to take shape to find out. Scientists, doctors and lay enthusiasts are investigating what could help or harm a baby even before that baby has been conceived. A few are now willing to make recommendations.

‮ ‬

Drug decisions before pregnancy

So far, only a few parents are aware of preconceptual clinics, books or advice. We have no idea how many actually do as they are advised. But even in these early days, prospective parents will find two types of advice to follow when it comes to decisions about drugs before pregnancy. Sometimes they are urged to be cautious. They need to be as careful of the drugs they take when they think they *might* be pregnant or might be pregnant soon, as they should be when they know they are.

Some advice for example suggests cutting down or avoiding alcohol altogether, although we still do not know the effect of maternal and paternal alcohol consumption prior to conception.

Other preconceptual advice takes the opposite tack, urging women, and, in some cases, men, to take *extra* drugs when preparing for pregnancy. This advice comes from both medical specialists and lay people, though more the latter. Their message is that, by taking drugs, you can improve the baby's chances of good health because you improve yourself. They usually recommend a combination of vitamins, minerals or trace elements and some suggest drugs to remove toxic chemicals from your body. A few enthusiasts even claim that all birth defects can be prevented by parental care and effort, but there is not much evidence to support such claims and the concomitant danger of creating anxiety and guilt if something does go wrong despite parental efforts.

Because these two approaches are so different, they deserve two chapters. The possible benefits of taking *more* drugs will be dealt with in the next chapter. This chapter will stick to the cases where caution is needed because of known risks, or where decisions need to be made because, inadvertently, you may have harmed your coming baby.

༉

The 'birth' of preconception

Everyone – parents and doctors – used to treat the first third of pregnancy fatalistically, and most still do. The standard approach for prospective parents was (and is) to wait, hope and see what happens. This explains why antenatal clinics only see women after ten weeks or so of pregnancy and why most books gloss over the topic. The detail and advice begins at about the time a woman registers with a medical authority and becomes officially pregnant. By then, it is too late to offer advice about the early weeks of pregnancy because most of the baby's organs have already formed (see Chapter 3).

Then along came in vitro fertilization and doctors could see, touch and manipulate eggs and sperm in order to oversee conception for their clients. New drugs, developed as adjuncts to IVF, will stimulate ovulation, prepare the uterus for implantation and even permit postmenopausal women to become pregnant. At the same time, a new way of managing diabetic women meant doctors could drastically reduce the chances that babies born to them would suffer malformation or harm. These were heady developments; they showed that things *can* be done to improve things for a tiny number of women, who no longer have only fatalism to fall back on. The hope is that it will be true for the rest. The myth is that this will happen soon.

Who knows how many forces might be at work or how many things could go wrong around conception? And which of the thousands of chemicals, drugs, diseases or habits that surround all of us might cause a problem? Fifteen years is a very short time to researchers keen to find answers to such questions. But it is a long time for prospective parents who see the door opening on the mysteries of conception, and who want firm recommendations about many things, including drugs. To do that, we will need many more studies and thousands more couples making various choices. While we wait for such studies, there are things you can do that are unlikely to cause harm and that are likely to increase the chances that your pregnancy and your baby will be as trouble-free as possible. The references for this Chapter include a range of leaflets and publications containing practical advice about planning a healthy pregnancy.

ᢒ

Dangers to egg, sperm and embryo

As far as drugs are concerned, the risk of a particular drug for the baby or the baby-to-be depends on when either parent takes it. Until conception, both parents are important in determining the baby's future prospects. Most of what we know about harm to egg or sperm comes from animal studies, though IVF techniques mean we are learning fast about humans.

Risks to the egg

When a girl is born, her body contains all the eggs she will ever produce. They are vulnerable to harm throughout childhood, though only a few substances are accepted hazards: radiation and anti-cancer drugs are the most commonly cited.

DRUGS TO AVOID BEFORE CONCEPTION

These drugs carry the specific recommendation that a woman should avoid pregnancy for some time after taking them.

Drug	Condition Treated	Waiting Time
Etretinate	psoriasis	Two years
Isotrinitron	acne	Three months
Danazol	endometriosis	Three months
	'morning	
	after pill'	
Penicillamine	rheumatoid arthritis	until blood tests
	toxic chemicals	normal

Eggs become more vulnerable to damage as each one ripens and bursts into the fallopian tube, ready to be fertilized. This takes a month or so for each egg, during which time extra vigilance is prudent. A drug that could damage the egg, taken in the month before pregnancy, could cause harm in three ways: it could prevent the egg from ripening at all, in which case the woman would not conceive; it could delay ripening which, in animals, has been linked with more abnormal eggs; it could change the egg itself which would probably greatly increase the risk of miscarriage.

Risk for sperm

The sperm that penetrates an egg and begins a new life, started its development about four months earlier. Only one in millions and millions is successful so nature has set the odds against abnormal sperm very high indeed. Nevertheless, some congenital abnormalities originate in the father rather than the mother. Men planning for a pregnancy are advised to consider the consequences of any drugs taken up to four months before conception. If specific dangers to sperm are known, the instructions with the drug should list any, but this is very rare.

Alcohol and smoking both increase the number of abnormal sperm (and one study has shown sperm concentration in smokers to be 24 per cent lower than in non-smokers).

Although it is possible to say that many things are detrimental to sperm formation, we cannot confirm that drug A caused abnormality B in a baby. Indeed, some drugs which are designed to harm sperm seem to have little effect on the baby. For example, in a study of 462 women who became pregnant whilst using spermacides for contraception, no increase was found in the number of abnormal children above that found in non-users.

The risk to the embryo

The chances of a baby being *born* damaged by something that happened between conception and around the time you miss your first period are low. Any damage will increase the risk of miscarriage, but, should one occur, it will not explain why it happened, as any number of causes are possible.

ॐ

Particular drug risks before pregnancy

Fertility drugs

Studies into the health of babies born to mothers taking clomiphene (Clomid), a commonly prescribed fertility drug, show a possible link with birth defects. That does not mean the drug causes the defect; it means that mothers who take Clomid have a slightly higher risk of delivering a baby with something abnormal. Most women who undergo fertility treatment find the desire to have a baby so powerful that it outweighs any slight risks.

Oral contraceptives

There are dozens of brand names and drug combinations, all referred to as the Pill. The active ingredients in your particular Pill will be synthetic oestrogen, synthetic progesterone (called progestogen), or a combination of the two. The packet information will show the constituents of yours.

It is not uncommon for a woman to keep on taking the pill without realizing she is pregnant. The risk of resulting abnormalities is very small, estimated at between one in 500 and one in 2000, and appears to be more likely to affect more babies. Progestogen-only pills seem to carry no increased risk to a baby but of course, the minute you think you might have conceived, you should stop the pill and use a barrier method until you know for sure that you are. In very high doses, such as the injectible contraceptive, Depo-provera, there is an increased risk that a girl baby's genitals will develop abnormally. One study found that the risk was around 0.07 per cent. That means that in 20,000 women taking the drug, you would expect to see an extra seven girls with abnormal genitals compared with the daughters of 20,000 who did not take the drug. The same study found a slight increase in the number of

PRE-PREGNANCY TASKS CONCERNING DRUGS

These are suggestions that continue to be prudent throughout life and can certainly be adopted at any point in pregnancy. You might want to discuss them at a preconception clinic, or with your doctor, if he or she understands and is interested in preconception.

- Check the medicine cabinet and throw away outdated medicines, old prescriptions and mysterious potions.
- Make a list of the drugs you take in a typical month. Be sure you include things you might not think of as drugs: vitamin pills, caffeine, cough medicine, aspirin, marijuana, tonics, etc. Then look in this book, ask a pharmacist or consult your doctor about what effect (if any) each drug might have on a developing baby.
- Keep a drink diary for a month. Record how much alcohol you drink in a week, and the maximum you drink at any one time. Once you have a total, look at it carefully. Though it could seem fine for you, it could be too much for your baby-to-be (see Chapter 12 for more information). Now is the time to plan how to cut down.
- If you are a smoker, assess how much you smoke a day, as this will tell you the increase in risk your baby will run should you continue (see Chapter 13). Then think hard about stopping. Giving up may be the single most helpful thing you can do for your baby. Have you really tried to stop? Have you tried hard enough?
- Reassess the contraception you are using. Most experts recommend women taking oral contraceptives stop at least three months before attempting to become pregnant. You will need to use some barrier method in the meantime. See page 43 for the possible consequences for the baby if the mother continues to take the Pill after she becomes pregnant.
- Never accept medications from other people – someone else's half finished course of antibiotics or headache tablet needs to be assessed as carefully as something in your own medicine cabinet.
- Tell any doctor, dentist, or X-ray technician that you might be pregnant even if you are not sure, so they can adjust your treatment accordingly.
- See your dentist and have any fillings done that might soon need attention.

Note: The Maternity Alliance and other organizations publish useful pamphlets on preconception (see page 253).

limb deformities in children born to mothers taking injectible contraceptives. Girls born to mothers taking synthetic oestrogens for other reasons, such as menopause treatment, or severe acne, have a 0.3 per cent risk of abnormal (too masculine) genitals.

༃

Summing up the case for preconception

We all know women who have ignored every suggestion offered and had a healthy baby. And we know women who have taken every precaution and then had difficulties. Neither is surprising once you consider how complicated the field of preconception is and how recently we have started to explore it. What should you do?

Each couple must find their own answers, usually starting with, 'What do you *want* to do?' Most then approach pregnancy in very much the same way they approach the rest of their lives (as the quotes at the beginning of the chapter show). It might help to look carefully at the consequences of their choice before making your own.

What about the first couple's approach – active planning? We cannot yet say that their efforts will benefit their baby but the evidence that certain actions seem to help and probably do no harm is growing. They are probably only a tiny fraction of the suggestions that will, in time, emerge as significant. Taking this course may well help the baby's chances of good health; they will not guarantee it.

And what of the second couple? Are they wrong to overlook the efforts of 15 year's work and research? Probably not. Most preconceptual advice is synonymous with recommendations for good health for all of us. What makes you strong, fit and happy is what is most likely to make your baby that way, too. They are already trying to do that.

And finally, what of the parents who suddenly discover they are pregnant? Not all will look back and feel good about the care they gave their child before they realized they were pregnant, because many of us have habits that risk our own and our children's health. Sadly, a few who feel this way will have babies who are unhealthy or abnormal. In only a tiny number of these cases will any firm evidence link what the parents did around conception with the outcome of the pregnancy.

৵

Decisions after taking drugs known to be dangerous

It could happen that, with hindsight, either parent feels they put the baby's health and wellbeing at risk by something they did or took around the time of conception. If you feel and judge the risk to be serious, you will need to think hard about what to do next. The choice is usually between carrying on with the pregnancy and seeking a termination. Neither is an easy option but parents grappling with the choices do seem to find that some things help them decide. They can also help parents live more easily with the consequences of their decisions.

Carrying on

If you choose this option, the most helpful thing you can do for your baby is to look after him or her the best you can during the rest of your pregnancy. This is easier said than done, of course, as one woman acknowledged when she told me of her own rocky start to pregnancy:

> You feel guilty when you look back and think 'I did this …
> I did that before I knew about the baby'. I felt horrible
> about it, a sinking feeling even though people kept saying
> it wasn't my fault. Now I realize that nobody can live their
> whole life always thinking, 'I could get pregnant by

mistake.' It would be like always thinking 'I could fall under a bus today.' But I worried every day for the whole pregnancy, until Jamie was born and was all right. I'd say to another woman who was in the same boat to concentrate on what you can do to help the baby. What's done is done. But I know she'd worry just like I did.

There are things you can do because they are good for babies, even those exposed to some risk. All the measures that make you more healthy will help. You could stop smoking because that's sure to help. You could learn relaxation techniques and find someone who will listen to your worries. Both of these will decrease the amount of stress hormones you transmit to your baby. And you could, as every parent must, remind yourself that tomorrow is another day … a phrase that has kept me going for over a decade.

Planning for a termination

Some people simply decide that carrying on with the pregnancy will be too difficult; others need help making up their minds. There are many agencies and counsellors who can help you make this very difficult decision, but they cannot be expected to know all the facts about risky drugs. You will help them do their job better (should you consult them), if you find the answers to a few questions first.

- How great are the risks? A handful of substances are dangerous enough to damage most of the babies exposed to them. A few dozen drugs, of the tens of thousands around, are known to harm a percentage of babies exposed. Many doctors would consider that inadvertent exposure to some, though not all, of the teratogens listed on page 20 would be grounds for termination should the parents so wish.

A few drugs will increase the risk of abnormality very slightly. You need a measure of how much more risk there might be in order to know what to do next. To find out: ask a pharmacist; see your doctor; read this book; get in touch with a self-help organization like those listed at the back of the book; or do all these things. The answers you get will vary a great deal. One woman was satisfied when a doctor said, 'You probably won't have a damaged baby.' Another located a government-funded drug advice service (see page 260) that told her that 38 studies, combined, gave a risk of 3.7 per 10,000 births in her particular case. Do keep asking until you find an answer that satisfies you.

- When did you take the drug? If the drug carries a specific risk of abnormality, did you take it at the time that that organ was still developing (see Chapter 3)?

- What particular abnormalities are connected with the drug and how do you feel about them? Only you can judge what you can or cannot cope with; only you know how the possibility of such a problem could fit in your life. One woman, on being told her baby might have a cleft palate, could be devastated. Another could feel like the epileptic mother who knew her necessary drugs increased the risk for her child and told me, 'Cleft palate isn't all that bad.'

- Is it possible to determine whether or not a potential problem is present? Some drugs are linked with specific abnormalities and, sometimes, it is possible to tell before birth whether or not the baby is affected. A good operator using high resolution ultrasound can spot limb deformities, heart defects and even some cleft palates, from about the sixteenth week. Some central nervous system deformities will produce an abnormal alfafoetal protein blood test. Some might be visible with a fetoscope. Having more information could make the decision easier, though, of course, the longer you wait the more traumatic the termination might be.

- How much does this particular pregnancy mean to you? I have been amazed over the years how much this varies between couples. I have heard of a couple who terminated an unplanned pregnancy because of a bit of beer drinking around conception. Another tried for years to get pregnant and when told that the ultrasound suggested the baby had a heart defect simply said, 'Hopefully, it can be fixed'. Only *you* can say how much this particular baby and this particular pregnancy means.

• Would it help to contact a specialist support group like SAFTA (Support After Fetal Termination)? They have helped many parents before and after terminations (see page 256).

ↄ

The basic message

Most pregnancies end in the birth of a live, healthy baby. Most of the time, the way we live is good enough and safe enough. Nevertheless, we owe it to our children to be prudent when we are warned of danger, and to use what knowledge we have to start their lives off as well as we can. To that end, the next chapter discusses whether extra drugs could bring this closer to reality.

ॐ 7 ॐ

Preconception – Going Beyond Risk Avoidance

The last chapter on preconception might have struck you as remarkably like all the health education you've been hearing all your life – 'Don't smoke', 'Don't drink too much', 'Don't take unnecessary pills', 'Look after yourself'! Advice about risk avoidance and tips about good health can leave some parents dissatisfied: 'Is that it? Is that all preconception has to offer?' This chapter is about where the dissatisfied might look for more in their search for what's best for themselves and their anticipated babies. Some of what it contains continues to be relevant right through pregnancy.

There are several reasons why parents want to know more than just how to avoid risks. Articulate and educated people are used to feeling in charge of their lives and they want the same when they decide the moment is right to start a baby. They feel unhappy leaving something as important as parenthood to chance. Other parents want to cover all the angles, hoping all will be well, but reasoning that some extra effort couldn't hurt. A third group seek preconception advice after a miscarriage, a complicated pregnancy or an abnormal baby. They want to know not only 'Why did it happen?' but also, 'How can we make sure it doesn't happen again?' And some people turn to preconceptual care either when they cannot conceive or cannot conceive fast enough.

These parents have many choices when it comes to preconceptual advice – they can consult people interested in everything from their psychic aura to their zinc levels. One suggestion parents might be given is that more drugs might improve their chances for a healthy and happy pregnancy. The most commonly mentioned ones are:

- *vitamins*
- *minerals* (calcium, chromium, copper, fluoride, iodine, iron, magnesium, potassium, phosphorus, selenium, sodium, and zinc).
- *trace elements* (less well known elements found in tiny amounts e.g. molybdenum)
- *and chelating agents* (drugs used to remove poisons like lead, mercury, arsenic and copper from the body. Penicillamine is the one most commonly cited)

It may seem strange to refer to vitamins and minerals as 'drugs' in this context. You may not have thought of them in this way because they are part of the food we eat. However, taken separately, in concentrated amounts or as single chemicals, vitamins and minerals are just as much drugs as any prescription you get from a doctor.

This chapter reviews the arguments for and against the idea that such drugs might help. Experts – both medically-trained and lay enthusiasts – take sides and argue passionately about this. Parents, too, find that these matters are not just part of an intellectual debate but touch deep feelings within themselves. Beneath parents' logical queries about zinc levels and the effects of aspirin, most harbour unspoken questions like, 'Am I healthy enough to have a normal baby? Am I fit enough? And if I'm not, how can I make myself good enough to do so?' Nothing I found while researching this book offers the answer to all these questions, nor do I believe we ever will be able to do so. What you can do is explore the different approaches on offer when it comes to extra drugs before pregnancy; only you can tell the one that best fits your other beliefs and values.

ॐ

The debate begins – is diet the key?

People are interested in food and supplementary vitamins and minerals before and after pregnancy, because many believe that diet is intricately connected with good health; it follows, they say, that it is equally important in pregnancy. Are parents correct to presume a connection between diet and pregnancy outcome? In the past few years there has been increasing interest in mothers' nutritional status before as well as during pregnancy in relation to birth weight and possibly the health of babies later in life. One study has suggested, for example, that babies who are small at birth (not preterm) may have increased rates of cardiovascular disease and non-insulin dependent diabetes as adults.

Could the food we eat also hold the clue to why things go wrong for the baby at the start of life and, if so, could we change the outcome by changing what we consume? Could it even be that too many or too few vitamins and minerals are the key factors in most birth defects?

Unravelling the answer is a bit like playing Pass the Parcel at a children's party – each answer leads on to the next question and explanation, and through it all, the arguments for and against extra vitamins and minerals continue. The role of diet is still a matter of uncertainty and controversy, and for most dietary interventions there have been few large enough studies to draw firm conclusions. The best place to begin exploring the issue is with four statements on which all experts agree:

1 *Women who are grossly deficient in certain vitamins and minerals are more likely to have babies who suffer congenital defects or poor health.* For example, women who have a genetic disease that makes them unable to absorb and use vitamin A, give birth to grossly abnormal babies. When these women take supplementary vitamin A, their babies are at no greater risk than any other. Animal studies have shown the same thing for nearly all vitamins and minerals – a diet that provides *no*

particular element results in high rates of death and deformity in the offspring.

2 *Pregnancy increases the requirements for most vitamins and minerals.* A new baby, a placenta, extra blood supply, more uterine muscle, extra fat stores – all can come only from what the mother eats or has already stored in her own body. To meet the new needs, she will need more of all the essential components of her diet.

3 *Some babies are at risk of poor health or abnormality because of their mother's diet.* Severe deficiency and malnutrition are very rare in Western countries but certain categories of women are more likely to be severely deficient in essential vitamins and minerals. These include: anorexics, adolescents, women having several children close together, alcoholics, drug addicts, and those with chronic illnesses. Some women are at risk of deficiency in some of the essential dietary components. For example, women who live on very low incomes often lack enough calories to meet the energy needs of pregnancy. Women who smoke, and those taking oral contraceptives, are often low in zinc and vitamin B_6. Nightworkers and some Asian women whose clothing leaves little exposed skin are low in vitamin D and may need supplements to achieve the current recommended intake of 10 mg/day. Strict vegetarians and vegans may be low in vitamin B_{12} and may need to increase their intake. They all need special diets and supplements do have their place in pregnancy if a need has been established.

4 *Some babies are more vulnerable to harm from deficiencies than others.* About 20 per cent of all birth defects occur because something triggers a tendency present in the genetic code, inherited from either the father or mother. This happens only in the babies who have inherited the tendency and then only in some of them. No one has any idea how to spot this sub-category of vulnerable babies. They are also not sure what these 'triggers' might be. There is some evidence (reviewed below) that deficiency of specific vitamins or minerals could be one such trigger.

Periconceptional folic acid supplementation can substantially reduce the risk of neural tube defects (such as spina bifida). The following section explains about this in more detail.

ॐ

Folate supplements

Folate known to reduce a particular vitamin called folic acid increase the risk of central nervous system (CNS) abnormalities, sometimes called neural tube defects (NTDs). The most common fetal malformations relate to NTDs and one of these, spina bifida, is four times more likely in some areas and in some social classes than in others. Doctors have long suspected that this reflects a variation in diet. To test their suspicions researchers gave women who had previously had a baby with a NTD multi-vitamins containing folic acid before their next pregnancy. The result was a striking fall – of two thirds – in abnormal babies. Several later studies also came to the same conclusion and others showed that taking folic acid supplements reduced the risk of NTDs in babies of women who had an affected pregnancy by 60 per cent. The latter is important because most NTDs occur in babies of women who have no history of such defects. It is now agreed by all the experts that folic acid supplementation pre-conception and up to the twelfth week of pregnancy (sometimes called periconceptional) can substantially reduce the risk of NTDs.

Other studies have also suggested that taking periconceptional multi-vitamins including folic acid can also reduce the risk of cleft palate and congenital abnormalities of the urinary tract, although the evidence for this is less strong and it is not clear whether the folic acid or one of the vitamins or the combination of all of them is responsible.

The Department of Health advises all women planning a pregnancy to increase their intake of folic acid. Specifically, women who have previously had an affected pregnancy should take 4 mg per day from the time they start trying to get pregnant until the twelfth week of pregnancy. Other women who have not had a problem with NTD before are advised to take 0.4 mg a day of folic acid supplement for the same period of time. Increasing the amount of folate in your diet is also recommended. Foods which contain folate include green leafy vegetables such as spinach, green beans, cauliflower, brussels sprouts, and milk, nuts, oranges and orange juice, pulses and yeast extract. Some foods such as breakfast cereals and certain breads are fortified with extra folic acid and you could check the contents labels of the ones you usually eat. There has been some debate about whether it is possible for women to get enough folic acid through diet alone. A recent study concluded that just eating folate rich foods may not be enough, and to be sure you should take extra folic acid as supplements and in folate fortified foods.

But remember, you can have too much of the good thing, and taking supplements at the recommended level and eating a folate rich diet is enough. Too much folate may interfere with the intake of zinc. Women who are taking drugs to control their epilepsy also need to be careful as it is thought that folate may reduce the effectiveness of these drugs.

Of course many women do not know that they are pregnant until it is too late for folate supplementation, but if there is a chance that you might become pregnant it would be worthwhile looking at your diet and increasing your intake of folate rich foods or switching to fortified cereals and bread.

Having agreed so far, pre-conception experts go their separate ways. The rest of this chapter describes each of these 'separate ways' in more detail.

ॐ

The 'good food only' advocates

If this chapter was a formal debate, in one corner would sit the mainstream, clinically-minded doctors who recommend that, with the exception of folate and women with special needs you do nothing more than follow a good diet before and during pregnancy. If you wish, you could take a daily multivitamin pill as long as it has been approved for use by pregnant women. (Read the label or packet insert to see if it is.) The multivitamin supplement is merely a 'belt-and-braces' move, unlikely to do any harm, possibly covering any deficit from the food you eat, and probably helping the parents feel satisfied that they are doing their best.

Unless there is clear clinical evidence (see above, numbers 1 and 3), these cautious doctors can offer good reasons for refusing to advise anything other than the diet you will find in any pregnancy book. Here are a few arguments in favour of 'good food only' for normal, healthy people and all those with no specific worries:

- worry about causing imbalance – We only understand the rudiments of how our bodies absorb, use and store nutrients, but we have established beyond doubt that the whole system is interconnected – change one bit of the system and the impact will be felt elsewhere. If you give more of one component (iron, for example) that may decrease the absorption of another (in this case, zinc). Changes in the amount of zinc absorbed will affect copper levels; and so on. The best way to be sure that mothers and babies get what they need is through a balanced diet, not concentrated supplements.

- worry about getting it wrong – The record of past efforts to manipulate diet for the benefit of mothers and babies has been patchy at best. Some interventions seem ineffective, like those of a well-known American obstetrician, Dr Thomas Brewer: he wrote books about diet and pregnancy that have a worldwide readership; he also runs a clinic for pregnant women where his ideas are put into practice. Yet when researchers compared mothers who did and did not attend the clinic, they found no relationship between attendance and low birth weight, prematurity or the number of babies who died between the twenty-eighth week of pregnancy and first week of life. 'Brewer' babies were not better off.

Other 'good ideas' turned out to cause more harm than good. When women on low incomes or state support were given extra protein and calories in the form of a dietary supplement, supplemented women had, on average, babies that weighed 32 grams *less* than controls who were not 'helped' in this way. The former babies were also more likely to be born too early and more likely to die in the first week of life. This finding was not unique. Another study found that high protein/low calorie supplements produced, on average, babies that were 400 grams lighter than the ones similar in every way except that their mothers took no supplements.

Interventions with specific vitamins and minerals have not always been helpful either. For decades, all pregnant women were prescribed supplementary iron and many still are. After reviewing 17 trials of the practice, one author could find no benefits in blanket iron prescriptions for healthy well-nourished women. (There is, however, a good case for iron supplements in cases where need is demonstrated, as explained on page 78.) It could even be that more harm was caused by upsetting zinc absorption than benefit offered to women who didn't need extra iron in the first place. Iron supplements can also cause heartburn, nausea, constipation or diarrhoea.

These and other experiences should deter the over-enthusiastic from prescribing supplements before they are proven effective by well controlled trials.

- uncertainty about how much to prescribe – Until we know how much of everything pregnant women need, we cannot determine the correct amount of supplements to prescribe. Every country publishes minimum daily requirements for most components in our diet – vitamins, minerals, protein, fats, carbohydrates. These vary a bit from country to country and the grounds for establishing minimums are obscure. An English obstetrician, writing an editorial on the subject for the *British Medical Journal*, tried to discover who set the UK minimums. The relevant government department told him it was 'a group of experts', using unexplained data at some point in the past. The vague answer makes assessing their validity impossible.

Many of us do not eat the right foods in the right amounts to achieve even minimal requirements. One Canadian study found that 37 per cent of women consumed less than three-quarters of the amounts recommended as a minimum, and 12 per cent consumed less than half. Yet most of these women will have normal babies and others whose diet is not deficient will not. Until we understand what women need, how much they need, and the consequences of having less than the recommended minimal amount, we must be cautious about interfering or advising women to do anything other than eat well.

⌇

The dangers of too many vitamins

Alongside the arguments just offered *in favour* of food is one *against* extra vitamins, especially large amounts of individual ones. Taking too much of some vitamins is dangerous for adults and very dangerous for growing babies. It can sometimes be difficult to convince people of this statement because of a widespread myth that vitamins can do no harm. They are 'good for you' and, if a bit is good, surely more is better and lots and lots are possibly very good indeed?

That's a question answered with a 'Yes' by many adults and a resounding 'No' by medical experts. Some people take tens or even hundreds of times more vitamins (and some minerals) than the recommended minimal amounts. This is called mega-vitamin therapy and pro-vitamin advocates base their argument on changes in the food we eat and the way we grow it. They believe that new ways of farming and processing food mean our diet doesn't contain the vitamins it otherwise would. Pollution and environmental toxins make our bodies less able to absorb and use the vitamins we do get. We need all the help we can get, they say, to stay healthy in a world that puts our bodies and minds under constant stress. Mega-vitamin therapy makes them feel better and stay healthier; health food shops are full of books that say the same.

Most adults can cope with mega-vitamin doses for varying amounts of time although the harm some cause must be balanced against the absence of any proof of benefit. Unborn babies are a different matter. The placenta actively moves vitamins in the baby's direction, in an effort to ensure the baby gets enough. Once in the baby, vitamins and minerals are hard to remove, Fat soluble ones (A and D) are stored in the fat and amounts that exceed the baby's needs build up to poisonous levels. Water-soluble vitamins (C and B_6, for example) and some minerals, are excreted via the baby's kidneys as they are in adults, but they only get as far as the amniotic fluid. The baby swallows and recycles them, adding to the supply from the placenta; levels continue to rise.

Once the baby's levels of particular vitamins reach an amount far in excess of the mother's blood levels, the baby is in danger. Except in a few rare cases where a genetic disease makes the mother unable to use and eliminate a particular vitamin or mineral, dangerous excess would only happen with mega-vitamin therapy. There are five particular dangers to watch out for:

- Vitamin A – This is a known teratogen in animals where researchers have demonstrated a clear association between high doses and birth defects affecting the eyes, brain and skeleton. There have been no reported cases of birth defects arising from excessive vitamin A intake in the UK, but cases have been reported from the USA and Spain where women taking mega-doses ranging from 6,000 microgrammes upwards have given birth to babies with deformities. Even clearer evidence is seen in women who took synthetic vitamin A as a drug (isotretinoin) to treat acne. They were 25 times more likely to have a deformed baby than matched controls.

  The recommended UK RDA is 2250 IU (750 microgrammes) of vitamin A. Vitamin supplements prescribed as part of antenatal care for pregnant women contain a safe amount of vitamin A. But many health food shops sell preparations including fish liver oil drops and tablets containing in excess of 25,000 IU/day, and one study found that 0.6 per cent of pregnant women were taking this amount daily. They will probably all have healthy babies, but they are, nevertheless, increasing the risk of harm without demonstrable benefit. (Because of the dangers of excess vitamin A the Chief Medical Officer has also advised against eating liver and liver products such as pâté – the vitamin A content of liver has increased in recent years and a 100g portion may contain 13,000–40,000 microgrammes.)

- Vitamin D – This is a fat soluble vitamin and accumulates in the baby when taken in doses over 400 IU/day. Too much vitamin D in animals causes high levels of calcium to build up in the baby's blood, leading to abnormal calcium deposits in the pups. Some human babies seem to be particularly vulnerable to this, while others can cope with very high levels without difficulty. Research on the subject records the birth of a normal baby to a woman who took 100,000 IU/day throughout pregnancy because of a disorder in her parathyroid gland. We have no way of predicting which babies are sensitive so restraint is recommended for all mothers. It is suggested that only groups of women who may be vulnerable to vitamin D deficiency because of poor diet or because their clothing exposes little skin to sunlight, or those with chronic illnesses which upset their body's ability to use vitamin D, should take extra. A dietician can recommend an appropriate dose.

- Vitamin C – Doses of vitamin C in animals lead to dependency in the offspring who metabolize and excrete the vitamin at a much higher rate than normal. At birth, when the supply is suddenly stopped, the pups develop scurvy, a deficiency disease caused by too little vitamin C. There are two cases of the same thing happening in human babies, one occurring after the mother took 400 mg/day throughout pregnancy. However, there appears to be no danger of tetratogenicity, based on animal studies. The recommended dose for pregnancy is 60 mg/day and the Department of Health has suggested increasing intake by 10 mg/day in the third trimester.

• Vitamin B_6 – Animal studies show no clear dangers from taking too much B_6 and many experts say they find no evidence of harm in humans. Others mention an increase in nerve abnormalities for babies exposed to high doses and say a state of dependency like that described above for vitamin C is a danger.

Judging what is 'too much' B_6 in pregnancy can be difficult as women are often recommended to take extra as a treatment for morning sickness, or to compensate for the lower levels associated with oral contraceptives. Unless a blood test confirms your levels are low, you are advised to increase your daily amount by only 0.6 mg/day in pregnancy, making a daily amount of 2.6 mgs/day. Discussion with your doctor would be prudent.

• Iodine – This is a teratogen in excessive amounts, leading to a goitre (enlarged thyroid gland) in the baby. There is no known case where this happened because of too much iodine in the ordinary diet but women who take kelp tablets (10–20 a day), use iodized salt, and iodized vitamins, are approaching the 'goitre' level.

Another source of iodine is cough expectorants so if you use them often you will need to read the label. Occasional use does not seem to pose a threat, however, as stated on page 112, there may be good reasons to reconsider the habit.

༄

The case for preconceptual supplements

Many people interested in diet and preconception would disagree with the 'good food only' advocates, viewing their approach as passive and overcautious. 'Tragedies do happen,' parents remind me, and I have never met parents who didn't worry about this. These feelings drive some people to making an extra effort before conception to try and ensure that they and their baby escape harm. They seek out advisers outside mainstream medicine who suggest many vitamin and mineral supplements to both improve their general health and eliminate toxins and poisons from their systems.

Implicit in this approach is the conviction that all abnormalities have causes and therefore they can be prevented. If this is so, parents hold within themselves the capacity to shape their baby's health and well being. An American academic, quoted in the booklet *Guidelines for Future Parents*, published by Foresight, the Association for the Promotion of Preconceptual Care (see page 253 for address), tells the reader (page 5), 'If human mates who are sound and capable of producing healthy offspring fail by producing malformed young, what more likely place shall we look for the fault than the developmental environment?' Taking up this theme, the booklet then suggests ways to improve yourself and, thereby, your baby-to-be. Following a section which describes, in detail, 16 vitamins and 13 minerals, the booklet's unnamed author concludes (page 42):

> By drawing attention to prospective parents to the tragic consequences of neglect of vitamin and mineral intake, we have not sought to frighten our readership to death! Rather, we have sought to reassure the average Parent-in-the-kitchen that the horrifying list of deformities and illnesses that can befall the baby in the womb are, in fact, not 'acts of God' which are entirely unavoidable, but that, to the contrary, most of them can be avoided very successfully ... You can easily skim down these pages and see what your body needs to build up a healthy and dare we say **perfect** [their emphasis] little baby! The remedy is available and not even on prescription ... a diet rich in these natural builders, stabilizers, cleansers and activators ...

Some parents find this reassuring and believe it to be, literally, life saving. In July, 1989, the *Observer* newspaper published just such a story. A woman describes four unexplained miscarriages which led her to give up trying to conceive because 'no explanation was given of our failure.' Then she heard of Foresight and there followed hair analysis for both partners, six months of vitamins and minerals, filtered water, dietary changes and more hair analysis. Finally, after costs which she said in the article came to £455, 'We were given the go ahead and were successful the first time.' She gave birth to a nine pound three ounce daughter.

You may read a story like that and wonder if such a regime would help you. The woman telling the story is convinced that her actions turned tragic 'failure' into 'success' and sees her baby as the proof. You could accept her conviction. But any obstetrician can cite cases of women who have had four miscarriages prior to the birth of a healthy baby without any special intervention. And you have no way of knowing how many other women followed the same regime and had a different outcome. To judge whether this woman's actions did indeed lead to her happy ending you need other evidence. The best evidence comes from large-scale trials where the parents who follow the regime are matched with other similar parents who are offered inert pills (placebos) instead of vitamins and minerals and chelating drugs. Ideally, neither the parents nor their doctors know whether the drugs used were the active or inert. In time, by comparing the parents who took extra drugs with similar ones who took a placebo, you would hope to see that the outcome for one set of parents is clearly better than that for the other.

Unfortunately, I could not find any reports of such studies for a regime like that described in the *Observer*, though the *Guidelines to Parents* does state: 'When we formed Foresight, we hoped we could substantially reduce the toll of miscarriage, perinatal death, congenital abnormality and very small babies. Happily, although numbers are small, this trend seems to be very clear.' If you take a broad range of supplements before pregnancy, you will do so out of a similar philosophical conviction that this approach *must* be helpful rather than from statistical evidence. Some parents will be wary, given the results of interventions like those cited in the section on better food rather than more supplements (pages 55–58) and the evidence for and against hair analysis (page 68). They are not happy with a 'try it and see' approach to general preconceptual supplements because the history of obstetrics is littered with instances where this was at best ineffectual and, at worst, actually harmful. Pro-vitamin groups point out that there is no evidence of physical risk from their regimes, with the exception of the five substances mentioned on pages 59–61.

As more studies are done, the question as to whether or not there are physical risks from taking extra supplements will become clearer; benefit, too, might be demonstrated. In the meantime, I have met parents who testify to emotional risks. Someone who knew I was thinking about preconception suggested I talk to Melanie. She had sought help after her second pregnancy went wrong and a course similar to the one already described was recommended.

> It was all about how I lacked this or did that wrong. Every week, the clinic doctor would ring with some new explanation about why the last pregnancy failed. Nobody seemed interested in me as a person, just how much magnesium or whatever was in my hair, and I felt I had to keep going until the numbers came back right. It was making me feel we'd never have another baby; I lost confidence in my body and myself. It took a good six months to begin to feel calmer after I stopped and over a year to conceive this baby. I personally know two other women who feel the same. Can I tell you more in a month or so? I'm due to have this baby any day and it's too upsetting to remember it all just now.

Four days later, she had a healthy little boy.

Pro-vitamin groups have the best of intentions and sincerely want to help parents. They recognize the pain of people like Pippa, who said, three months after her first baby was stillborn, 'I've spent days and nights wracking by brains for why it happened. All the tests were negative and I can't think of anything I did differently from all the other women in my antenatal class. Sometimes, I still go nearly crazy asking why, why, why ...'

In another Foresight booklet, *Specific Anomalies and Some Relevant Research*, the author agrees (page 5): 'To have a child born with a problem is sad. Not to be able to account for the cause is agony.' They are contacted by parents who cannot, like Pippa, live with her conclusion, 'Bloody bad luck.'

But I believe that it is no kindness to claim you can have perfect babies, or to lay the blame for imperfect ones on parents, until scientific evidence is much clearer than it presently is. When one American academic writes in the *Guidelines for Parents* (page 5), 'If we cannot yet control Nature, we do nevertheless have the means to control nurture,' he is expressing a dream for the future, not an assessment of present reality. If, and when, the dream of 'controlling nurture' comes true, then pain, guilt, blame and money would be costs many parents would willingly bear. Until it does, only you can judge if they are too high for you, as you prepare for pregnancy.

༄

Selective supplements in pregnancy

You may feel, after the last few pages, that neither of the above approaches suits you as you prepare for pregnancy. Doctors who advocate sticking to recognized dietary advice may sound complacent. How can we do nothing when there is so much evidence that things *do* go wrong? And lay enthusiasts who claim we can control our babies' health if we just try hard enough may strike you as either well-meaning cranks or disturbing fanatics. You may be wondering, 'Is there no other choice?'

The rest of this chapter reviews evidence that suggests that specific deficiencies may be important in predicting the health of your baby-to-be. Having too little or too much of specific chemicals could act as a trigger to cause otherwise dormant inherited defects. By finding out if you *are* deficient in one or the other substances known to be linked with defects, you might be able to lessen the chances that one particular defect develops. Remember, you can reduce the odds, but you can never eliminate the risk completely.

Zinc supplements

More research effort has gone into discovering the role of zinc in pregnancy than any other mineral. The results are intriguing but inconclusive. After reviewing hundreds of articles, one researcher summarized his findings as follows.

1 Adequate amounts of zinc are necessary for normal development and normal bodily function.
2 Severe deficiency leads to high rates of abnormality in animals and humans. Where genetic disease makes the mother unable to metabolize zinc, 43 per cent of the resulting babies are abnormal.
3 Some studies show intriguing connections between zinc level and pregnancy outcome. When researchers measure zinc levels in babies who have abnormalities, or mothers who have experienced serious pregnancy complications, they do find them lower than those of unaffected babies or mothers. It is thought that low zinc levels may cause heart defects and growth retardation. Intervention studies (these are studies where the doctor first diagnoses a zinc deficiency then gives women with lower than normal levels extra zinc) show an association between zinc levels and pregnancy outcome. In one study, supplemented women had fewer overdue babies and smoother, more effective labour contractions. Another showed fewer instances of pregnancy-induced hypertension in adult women (no change was seen in supplemented adolescents). Many more studies are currently underway to clarify the link between zinc and pregnancy outcomes.
4 Most diets fail to meet the recommended daily amounts for zinc.

The over-hasty would look at these four points and reach for zinc supplements, and they would get much encouragement from the pro-zinc lobby who call zinc 'The Super Mineral'. The more cautious would notice we lack several things usually considered vital before recommending general supplementation.

Overall there is a risk of consistency in study findings; the links with intrauterine growth retardation are uncertain; and the amount of zinc required is not clear. And the studies quoted above simply show that two things happened together (low zinc and complications); they do not show that one caused the other. That would not matter so much if a randomized control trial (RCT) showed that giving zinc helped women and babies more than doing nothing, and more than it harmed them. A recent RCT found that daily supplements given to women with *low* plasma zinc concentrations in early pregnancy improved infant birthweight. But this was a group of women with poor zinc status and who were at greater risk of having a low birthweight baby, and the results do not justify giving zinc supplements to every pregnant woman. Although no harm has been found in giving women who are known to be deficient extra zinc, we cannot justify doing so for everyone, until benefit has been shown to outweigh harm. The fact that animal studies have demonstrated that zinc supplements can harm and that intakes above 50 mg/day could cause copper deficiencies means that we should be restrained.

Would it make sense, then, to find out if you are one of the women who need more zinc, then take extra? Some groups are known to be deficient: these include anorexics, diabetics, alcoholics, those undergoing chelation therapy, those with chronic illnesses, and those who have recently had a serious injury or burn. Other groups *might* be deficient. Women taking contraceptives are said to have lower zinc levels. It also seems possible that taking folate supplements can reduce the body's ability to absorb zinc. Finding out one's zinc level is not straightforward – two kinds of tests are on offer – either a blood test or hair analysis – and each has its drawbacks.

A blood test could measure the amount of zinc in the plasma (the liquid component of blood) but less than 1 per cent of the total amount of zinc held in your body is found there; the rest is found in your cells. If you are already pregnant, you can expect a low reading because all zinc levels fall in pregnancy, reflecting perfectly normal changes in how our bodies absorb and use zinc.

Hair analysis involves sending a predetermined length of hair to a specialist laboratory, but the problems are legion. There is no established range of what is 'normal' and this makes judging the significance of numbers from the lab impossible. Results also vary according to the method used. An editorial in the medical journal, the *Lancet* describes sending identical samples to two labs and receiving conflicting results. Tests can be affected by various confounding factors, because if hair grows slower, chemicals concentrate. Some people claim contaminants like air pollution, swimming pools, and shampoo are a problem, and they will affect the analysis. Finally there are many very low readings with no apparent illness. When samples of young, healthy women are examined, about half the readings indicate that something is wrong but nothing is evident. Do we believe the hair over clinical evidence?

Those in favour of hair analysis say it is 'cheap, effective and non-invasive'; those against call it 'flourishing ... but useless, unscientific, economically wasteful, and possibly illegal'. If you turn to hair analysis as one way of assessing your mineral status, you are choosing an option not recognized by the medical profession as a whole, but nevertheless used by some. Only you can judge if it is reliable enough to justify taking extra minerals which, in excess, carry a risk for your baby.

If, on the basis of your own clinical history or tests, it seems that extra zinc is needed, it is very unlikely that diet alone is enough to make up the deficit. Generally diet only supplies between a third and a half of the recommended daily amount (RDA) for pregnancy of 20–30 mg/day. Since most mothers and most babies are fine despite this continual shortfall, we can only presume that the RDA is set too high.

Good sources of zinc include liver, beef, cheese, milk, sardines, oysters and shrimp and even if they will not ensure you reach the over-ambitious RDA, non-vegetarians will eat well trying! Vegetarians need to eat more nuts, wholemeal bread and yeast which contain zinc.

Women who feel in good health and who are confident that their diet is adequate should feel little need to take extra zinc before or during pregnancy. Those already pregnant who did nothing about their zinc levels have no cause for worry unless they fall into the category of women known to be at risk. If they are at risk, the chances are that they will be ill enough to have already consulted a doctor and discussed the whole range of nutrients they lack.

Parents who choose, despite the ambivalent evidence, to supplement their zinc levels may or may not be helping their children – we await further research with interest before we can say for sure.

Copper

Copper has only been shown to be lacking in areas of the world where it is deficient in the soil and thus lacking in crops (for example, a large area of China). There is little chance that your baby will be short of copper because he or she can store most of what is passed through the placenta, and food sources are widely available. A further argument against supplements is the known toxicity of copper – too much is very bad for babies.

Fluoride

Five studies on the influence of fluoride all show a decrease in the dental decay of the babies born to women who took fluoride supplements. There is no evidence of any harm to the pregnancy or to the baby although it is not clear whether taking fluoride supplements is a good idea if you live in an area with high levels of fluoride in the water. Tooth formation starts around the fourth month of pregnancy and there is little to be said for taking it before this time.

Other Minerals

Two minerals – iron (see page 78) and calcium – are important for healthy pregnancies and babies. A systematic review of controlled trials (in 1994) of calcium supplementation shows promise of reducing pregnancy–induced hypertension and pre-eclampsia but there is insufficient evidence to recommend routine supplementation, and not enough is known about safety. Similarly, recommendations to take magnesium supplements during pregnancy are not backed up with any concrete evidence.

⟱

The case for and against supplements

I feel uncomfortable when I read, as one doctor wrote in a book about preconception aimed at normal, first-time parents:

> In the same way an athlete strengthens her body to run a gruelling marathon, a woman can ready her body [for] pregnancy … you may also be training your fetus for a better start in the marathon of life.

This is not just a recipe for exhaustion (I do hope this dynamic mother lets her newborn sleep now and again) but for fantasy, too. We cannot make everything all right if we just work hard enough. Sometimes, in trying to do so, we can even cause ourselves and our babies harm, as one or two instances in this chapter illustrate. Unless we remember our limits, we take on too much responsibility when things go wrong.

What is not understood cannot be prevented, and almost everything in preconception is not yet understood. A good diet, stopping smoking and avoiding excess alcohol can all help to ensure that prospective parents are in good health prior to conception. But there is not enough scientific evidence to justify supplementation with vitamins and trace elements, with the exception of folic acid and, for some vulnerable women, vitamin D. Be wary of anyone who offers sweeping explanations or blanket guarantees. The curtain is starting to lift and offer tantalizing suggestions for the future. It could be that, when your own children have babies, they will have clearer answers to questions about what extra drugs might help mother and baby have a healthier, happier pregnancy.

PREGNANCY

✌ 8 ✌

Drugs Used For Acute Illnesses

It is estimated that about one in 20 women will get an infection illness during pregnancy. This chapter is about drugs prescribed by doctors for acute illnesses, this includes any illness that comes on quickly and, with the appropriate treatment, will be cured quickly.

Illness that comes on slowly, lasts a long time (possibly even all your life), and has no cure though drug treatment can make the symptoms less troublesome or dangerous, is called chronic illness. Drugs for these conditions are described in the next chapter.

If you are *not* pregnant and fall ill, your choices are fairly clear cut. You could ignore it – most illnesses do go away by themselves – or you could take a few aspirins and go to bed. Advertisements have been recommending you do this all your life. Or you could ask a doctor to diagnose the problem and, in the majority of cases, accept a prescription that will alleviate the symptoms, or do away with the underlying cause. Any or all of these actions are appropriate but once you are pregnant or even think you might be, what do you do if you fall ill?

Suddenly, there are new rules and new assumptions about how to handle illness. Your baby, too, is involved in the consequences of what you decide. Whatever decision you make, there are some preliminary assumptions that will always apply.

If it is possible to avoid drugs, that is the counsel of perfection. You will need to weigh up the consequences of *not* taking something as carefully as you might consider taking it.

Any drug you take will reach your baby. Long gone are the days when we imagined the baby was like a tiny astronaut, isolated from the world and safe in a sheltered capsule. If a drug enters your bloodstream, it will reach your baby. The time it takes to do so varies – some drugs cross the placenta quickly, while others take many hours. The amount of the drug that crosses varies too – some drugs reach concentrations in the baby which are the same as the mother, or which are even greater, while others cross with difficulty and only a trace reaches the baby. The effects vary too. A few harm the developing baby, most seem to have a neutral effect, and a handful are given specifically to benefit the baby as well as the mother (for example heart drugs for a baby's abnormal heart rhythms diagnosed before birth).

Any effect the drug might have will depend on the stage of development that the baby has reached. At some stages of development, a baby is more vulnerable to the effects of drugs than others and in order to know what the effect *might* be, you need to know what stage of development the baby has reached (see Chapter 3).

$\mathcal{D}$

Asking for a prescription drug

As already stated, the number of babies actually damaged by the drugs or chemicals that their mothers took in pregnancy is very small – only around 1 per cent of all congenital handicaps requiring major surgery, or posing a threat to a baby's life and well being, can be traced to anything the mother took. The list of drugs *known* to cause birth defects is also small (see page 20). The list of known teratogens is far from secret knowledge but you are advised not to take your doctor's vigilance for granted. It is always a good idea to inform any doctor you see that you are contemplating pregnancy from the moment you cease contraception. Some women even state that they are in the second half of their menstrual cycle, and could be pregnant.

That way, both of you will be aware that a potential baby, too, is part of the decision as to what kind of treatment is best.

'Treatment' need not, of course, always mean drugs. Indeed, in many cases, drugs are not the answer at all. Some problems have no effective drug treatment. A dose of flu – caused by a virus and thus unresponsive to antibiotics – will go away in its own time. Even though the risk of teratogenic damage is very small for antibiotics (the older ones have been used for decades without any noticeable harm), it is not worth even this small risk as they offer no benefit for viral illnesses.

Some problems can be treated by other forms of treatment besides a prescription drug or even an over-the-counter remedy. Constipation, for example, can be helped by changing your diet. Anxiety is less of a problem if the sufferer learns relaxation techniques. Easing backache is the stock-in-trade of obstetric physiotherapists – you might try them before you consider drugs. Many women turn to alternative therapies as described in Chapter 11.

Some infectious illnesses such as syphilis and toxoplasmosis which can cause congenital defects can and should be treated. Syphilis can be treated with antibiotics, toxoplasmosis can be safely treated with spiramycin although it is uncertain how effective this is. And for Chlamydia, which may be associated with intrauterine growth retardation and premature labour, the WHO recommends erythromycin.

However, a decision to opt for a prescribed drug to treat most acute illnesses in pregnancy should be preceded by careful thought unless the benefits are obvious. Before you seek such help, it might help to ask yourself these questions: Is there likely to be a drug treatment that will help me get better quickly? What are the likely effects on my baby of accepting such treatment? What are the effects for me and my baby of doing nothing? What other options do I have?

The rest of this chapter describes acute illnesses that often coincide with pregnancy and require drug treatment.

༄

Anaemia in pregnancy

There are many different forms of anaemia and your doctor will offer the form of treatment appropriate to the particular anaemia diagnosed. By far the most common in pregnancy is caused by your body needing more iron than it can get from the food you eat or the stores in your body. Without enough iron, your body cannot make enough haemoglobin; too little haemoglobin means the red blood cells cannot carry enough oxygen; too little oxygen means you feel tired, faint and generally awful. Anaemic women are probably more prone to infection and more likely to bleed in childbirth. Their babies may be underweight and more likely to develop anaemia in the first year of life.

The way to treat this problem is with extra iron. This could come from a diet richer in foods higher in iron (liver, meat, eggs, leafy green vegetables, and pulses) or from iron pills or injections. Millions of women taking iron over decades have convinced doctors that iron is not teratogenic. On the contrary, there is evidence to suggest that women given iron have babies with fewer abnormalities, though the connection is not yet proven. However, taking iron supplements can be unpleasant as they cause stomach irritation.

The greatest danger associated with iron supplements is not to the woman herself but to other children who find the pills. Toddlers have died from accidental overdose.

Whether or not to take iron prophylactically (before you become anaemic in the hope you do not) is controversial. If your doctor suggests iron supplements before your blood tests show they are warranted, you could ask why you are at risk. A blanket prescription ('We like all our ladies to take extra iron …') without evidence of particular need would be out of step with current thinking by most doctors. Most women who are well nourished have sufficient iron stores to meet increased needs during pregnancy, and the body increases the uptake of iron from food during pregnancy. Supplementation is only necessary for those whose iron stores are low at start of pregnancy. (Women with sickle cell and thalassaemia often receive blood transfusions in pregnancy and iron supplementation should be avoided in case of possible iron overload.)

One author, reviewing the case for and against prophylaxis in the *British Medical Journal* in 1988, summed up the argument as follows:

> The point of antenatal care is to identify those at risk and to deal with the problem, and my own view is that wholesale supplementation is probably inappropriate and this is supported by BNF which advises against routine iron supplementation, and by a large number of recent studies.

꒰ꕤ꒱

Antibiotics in pregnancy

Ten per cent of pregnant women take antibiotics. If your doctor has diagnosed an infection that is likely to respond to an antibiotic, he will probably prescribe one. You will need as much medication for as long as you would when you are not pregnant; some women may even need more medication to get the same benefit.

Your doctor will have a wide range of antibiotics to choose from but he or she will probably stick to penicillin or ampicillin, which have been used for decades without any noticeable ill effects for the baby. Advice to doctors usually suggest these rather than newer variations for which no long-term information is available.

However, allergy to penicillin or ampicillin is always a possibility. If your baby is allergic to either drug, you are sensitizing him or her by taking the first dose and for that reason, a few doctors recommend a single large dose rather than a course that spreads over many days. Do mention the antibiotic that you have taken during pregnancy should you need another again or if your baby needs one after birth.

If you are allergic to penicillin/ampicillin, the next choice could be one of the sulphonamides. These drugs have an even longer track record than penicillins as they were developed in the 1930s. Again, no one can say for sure that they are safe, and sulphonamides have harmful side-effects near to the birth (they can cause the baby to be jaundiced if taken within two days of birth), but after 50 years of use, there have been no noticeable long-term effects on babies.

A few antibiotics should be avoided:

- tetracycline because it causes staining of milk teeth and abnormal bone development.
- streptomycin (and probably gentamycin and kanamycin) because they could damage the baby's hearing
- erythromycin because it could damage the mother's liver (though it may be used in some infections such as Chlamydia if the benefits balance or outweigh the risks)
- chloramphenicol because it can cause serious blood disorders in mother and baby.

Of course, these are only general recommendations. You may be allergic to some medications; some may be ineffective against the cause of this particular infection. Doctors may even prescribe drugs known to be dangerous in cases where the risk to the mother is great enough to justify the decision. Ann's story illustrates how decisions have to be made and remade as situations change.

I was terribly sick with both my pregnancies the whole way through. I remember watching the Cup Final on TV when I was pregnant with Hannah and being sick twenty-two times. I ended up in hospital with both of them because of dehydration. It was *awful*. When I was pregnant the second time the same thing happened and after eight weeks, my resistance was so low I developed encephalitis [an infection of the brain – often fatal and, in the form Ann had, known to be teratogenic]. I nearly died. They treated me with every IV drug in the book for about two weeks before it looked like I might make it. Then one day, a doctor I'd never met before came in and asked when I wanted the abortion. I was too weak to be angry but just strong enough to throw him out. I never saw him again. I knew that I would never go through another pregnancy and it was this baby or none and I just hoped the baby would make it. I was determined to give him the chance ...

Ann had to stop telling her story several times to deal with normal, demanding Jack, now aged four!

In this case, it was clear that Ann needed treatment. Other cases are less clear cut. However, it is usually best to treat:

- urinary tract infections (symptoms include burning or pain on passing urine; and an urgent need to empty your bladder) as they can lead to kidney infections and possibly, premature labour
- a sore throat if you also have a fever, swollen glands and fast heartbeat
- bronchitis that follows on after a heavy cold
- any irritation of the vagina that includes itching, redness, or foul-smelling discharge (see the next two sections for information about the usual drugs used)

✌

Antifungal drugs

Pregnancy changes the chemistry of your vagina and, to some extent, your mouth. When this happens, the yeast, Candida, which is normally present but does not cause any problems, can suddenly flourish. When it does, you have a thrush infection. Vaginal thrush is estimated to be between two and ten times more common in pregnant women than in women who are not pregnant. If the problem occurs in the vagina, you can get a thick, creamy discharge, itching and soreness. A vaginal swab will confirm the diagnosis after examination in a laboratory. Thrush in pregnancy is best treated with topical preparations (pessaries placed in the vagina to work directly on the fungus) rather than those taken orally. Imidazole preparations, such as micronazole (Gyno-Daktarin, Monistak), clotrimazole (Canestan) and econazole, are more effective than nystatin. Oral drugs such as flucazole have been tested in pregnancy and cannot be assumed to be safe.

Other antifungal drugs are given orally or intravenously for fungal infections inside the body. They would only be prescribed for pregnant women if her life was in danger.

ॐ

Antiprotozoan drugs

The last section described a vaginal infection (thrush) caused by the yeast, Candida. Less common, but equally in need of treatment, is the vaginal infection caused by the protozoan, Trichomonas. This organism causes a smelly, irritating vaginal discharge. If your doctor suspects trichomoniasis, he or she will take swabs and send them for identification. Treatment is less straightforward than for thrush. The drug choice (for both partners) is metronidazole (Flagyl). It has caused abnormalities in lab animals but a recent meta-analysis (review of several studies) which looked at 32 studies concluded that there was no increased risk of abnormalities from taking metronidazole during the first 14 weeks of pregnancy. However most doctors refrain from using it in early pregnancy to be on the safe side. You and your doctor will have to weigh up the risks in view of the severity of the infection and the stage of your pregnancy.

༄

Emergency operations and anaesthesia

There are no recorded ill effects from exposing babies to general anaesthesia in the first two-thirds of pregnancy. Most of the studies are retrospective – that is, looking back after the babies were born – and most are for small numbers. Lots of anecdotal evidence shows that babies can cope with general anaesthesia without harm. Like most doctors, yours can probably cite cases of women with appendicitis, gallstones, or even gunshot wounds, who then go on to have healthy children. Nevertheless, you should be sure the doctor or dentist knows you are or might be pregnant should a general anaesthetic be suggested for anything other than major surgery.

༄

High blood pressure caused by pregnancy

See pages 98–101

༄

Malaria in pregnancy

An acute attack of malaria is dangerous for the baby – it is associated with higher rates of miscarriage and premature labour. The fever, too, may be risky. If you are planning to go to an area where malaria is a possibility, you need good protection against the disease, starting one week before you go and continuing for four weeks afterwards. This is especially true in the last third of pregnancy.

Because the malaria parasite is becoming more and more resistant to some drugs, you will need to think carefully about the best one to ward off acute attacks. In some areas – notably East and Central Africa, South-east Asia, and South America –

the malarial parasites are resistant to the safer drugs. Many doctors feel that the risks involved in prescribing the drugs that are effective (Maloprim and Fansidar) are too great for pregnant women and advise them to avoid travel to these areas. Another alternative is to stay in cities and take chloroquine (see below) every week and proguanil (Paludrine) daily. Paludrine is said to have adverse effects only in large doses. Acute attacks should be treated with quinine.

In North Africa and the Middle East, the parasite is not resistant to chloroquine and this remains the best drug. Chloroquine has only been known to cause damage to the baby when given in very large doses, not in the amounts used to keep malaria at bay. You should avoid primaquine completely as it is known to cause serious blood disorders in the baby.

჻

Migraine in pregnancy

There are many reasons why you might have a migraine headache and the treatment will vary depending on the cause. How-ever, the drug of choice for a migraine headache in ergotamine. This is not prescribed in pregnancy because it causes the uterus to contract, increasing the risk of miscarriage in the early months, and premature labour later on.

჻

Nausea and vomiting in pregnancy

Debendox (also called Bendectin in North America) was used to treat 'morning sickness' nausea and vomiting for many years: as many as 33 million pregnant women took it between 1964 and 1983. It was described as 'highly successful' in reducing the symptoms of morning sickness yet the manufacturers withdrew it from sale in 1983. At that time, the company faced 250 court cases from American women who claimed the drug caused birth defects in their babies. The company settled these cases out of court, stating that this 'should not be construed as an admission of liability'.

Despite many studies, no firm evidence exists linking Debendox with birth defects in humans. Animal tests did show that the drug increased the number of deformed offspring. Women who took the drug did give birth to children with a variety of deformities but the kinds of deformities and the number affected were the same as for a matched population of women who *did not* take the drug. Scientists could not show that Debendox was a teratogen in humans despite very large studies (and there has been no reduction in the incidence of reported malformations since Debendox was withdrawn). But neither could they conclude that Debendox is definitely *not* a teratogen because proving a negative result is virtually impossible.

The result: caution prevailed and the drug was withdrawn to spare the company future expensive court cases. (We should be grateful that all manufacturers do not follow this line of reasoning for, as one expert points out, 'If we based practical decisions on experimental work alone, we would eliminate the vast majority of foodstuffs, medicines, household chemicals and petroleum products which are an integral part of our lives.')

By and large, women have to cope with nausea in pregnancy by non-pharmacological means. Two small randomized controlled trials have for example shown acupuncture to help in reducing persistent nausea. Other women have found hypnosis and acupressure helpful, and one study has reported on a RCT that showed vitamin B_6 therapy significantly reduced severe nausea and vomiting. Unless your sickness is severe enough to threaten your health – and that means very severe indeed – your doctor is unlikely to prescribe anything to ease it. If the symptoms are severe, you may be offered an antiemetic such as pyridoxine, meclozine, promethazine or prochlorperazine. These antihistamines are generally considered to be safe enough to warrant fairly widespread use for severe nausea. However, they do cause drowsiness and occasionally blurred vision, and there have been no major studies to assess potentially adverse effects on the baby. In late pregnancy, some doctors prescribe metaclapramide to ease constant nausea and vomiting or to prepare a woman for surgery. No evidence on how it affects the baby is known, so it cannot be recommended for use in early pregnancy.

❧

Summing up

It is not always better to grin and bear things. If something is causing you pain, talk to your GP. If some illness is not improving, seek help. It is in your baby's best interest that you are well and that may mean taking drugs to achieve a return to health.

Drugs For Chronic Conditions

When it comes to weighing up the risks and benefits of prescribing a drug in pregnancy, no choices are easy, as we saw in Chapters 4 and 5. But where chronic* illness coincides with pregnancy, women are faced with painful choices. In a few cases, the drugs that promote the mother's health are teratogenic. In all cases, the drugs cross the placenta and have some effect – not necessarily a harmful effect – on the baby.

At first glance, the decision seems to be 'Myself or my baby ...?', an agonizing choice made more terrible by Western cultural beliefs that mothers should always put their baby's needs first. On the surface, chronically-ill women appear to do the opposite. If you know someone struggling in this cleft stick or you yourself are doing so, it may help to remember that, by getting the right treatment, a mother not only helps herself but she is also doing something positive for her baby. That's true ... even though it does not always feel that way.

There are things that make choices easier for chronically-ill women. They and their offspring are 'interesting'. Some conditions have attracted hundreds of papers and research projects. Doctors have worked out drug regimes that seem to work, though, unfortunately, they seldom have the benefit of large-scale trials to test their ideas. But more studies are published all the time and knowledge is growing. Long-term

---

* 'Chronic' in this context means an illness that comes on slowly and lasts a long time.

follow-ups have also been done on the babies, so we have some idea of their continuing health. As a result, we do know a good deal about the risks and benefits of particular drugs.

If you are chronically ill, you are probably used to weighing up risk and benefit for yourself so you can do so more confidently than women who have never thought this way about drugs before. Hopefully, too, you have a long-standing relationship with the doctor caring for you which should make talking easier. If this is not the case, you may want to think about changing doctors because you are likely to see much more of each other in the pregnancy. Nearly all chronically-ill women need close monitoring and careful checks to make sure their drug requirements stay correct. If you do not feel the doctor you have is particularly interested in pregnancy or willing to offer you the support you deserve, this could be the time to find one who is. The organizations listed on page 253 may be able to help if you wish to change doctors.

჻

Making decisions

Every woman deserves time, information and support to help her make up her mind about drugs in pregnancy, and if you are chronically ill, you probably need even more of all three. The best time to start is before you are pregnant – months or even years before in some cases! That way, not only are you in the best shape possible to launch the pregnancy but you are also spared any worry about inadvertent exposure for your baby in the first few weeks of his or her development.

If you did not manage to sort out your drugs before becoming pregnant, it's important to do so as quickly as possible. You could ring up your doctor today and explain why you need an urgent appointment. There may be alternative treatments as effective as the drug regime you are presently following; or your condition could be one that improves during pregnancy (rheumatoid arthritis, for example). Because pregnancy changes how your body uses drugs and even alters the chronic illness itself, you will probably need new drug regimes.

It is almost never a good idea to simply stop taking whatever drugs you have. Your health could suffer and as a result, so could your baby's. In the case of drugs that cause dependency, like mood-altering drugs and drugs treating epilepsy, stopping abruptly could cause withdrawal symptoms. Ask for help from your doctor to reduce the dose gradually to zero if possible.

The descriptions that follow are only offered as suggestions for what you might want to discuss when you talk with your doctor. New information comes to light every week and you may need to take that into account, too.

⁊

Women with asthma

It appears that asthmatic women may experience an increase in respiratory symptoms when they are pregnant, although this may be because some stop their medication for fear of harming the baby. But, the evidence is that controlling the symptoms of asthma results in a pregnancy no more complicated than those of unaffected women. In fact you are more likely to harm your baby if you stop medication. The baby is at greater risk from a severe and uncontrolled attack than from medication used to control asthma. Studies of babies whose mothers have taken asthma drugs are also reassuring. One study of 145 babies whose mothers took steroids in the first twelve weeks showed they were no more at risk of damage than those of non-asthmatic mothers. Similar reassuring results were found when studying the babies whose mothers used an inhaler containing a beta-blocking drug like salbutamol. These are small studies and do not prove that there is no danger, but may imply that the danger, if any, is small.

Many of the medications used to manage asthma (beta antagonists, oral steroids, inhaled beclomethasone, methylxanthines) have been widely used for many years with no evidence of any tetarogenic effect. There is less experience with more recently introduced inhaled steroid budesonide and inhaled anti-cholinergic ipratnoprium but neither have been shown to be dangerous in pregnancy. Oral theophylline treatment has been suspected of causing malformations, and a recent study concluded that while moderate doses in the second and third trimester can be considered safe, safety in early pregnancy is less clear. Inhaled steroids act only in the lungs and little of the medicine is absorbed into the bloodstream. Steroid tablets act through the blood but do not harm the baby at doses of less than 45 mg/day.

About 1 per cent of pregnant women suffer from active asthma. Jackie does – she has taken steroids for 20 years, through three pregnancies, and denies any worry about the consequences of taking drugs. She says, 'If I don't, I just can't function.' Like 25 per cent of all asthmatics, her symptoms actually got worse in pregnancy (50 per cent say they noticed no change; 25 per cent said they were better in pregnancy).

Jackie's doctor probably feels the same confidence in his decision to treat her as she does. Studies of the effects of corticosteroids in pregnancy are small – 45 pregnancies in one case; 38 in another – but neither of these showed an increase in congenital malformation, miscarriage or neonatal death. Other studies have suggested that there may be a small increase in the risk of cleft palate and intrauterine growth retardation from corticosteroids. But, on the other hand, you need to remember that an acute asthma attack could deprive a baby of oxygen, something that is especially dangerous in the first 12 weeks.

If you have asthma, you will need to talk with your doctor about any changes to your current drug regime. A 1987 report in the *British Medical Journal* recommends: reducing the number of drugs taken to a minimum; cutting out antihistamines; using inhaled bronchodilators (salbutomol and terbutaline appear safe); using a spacer device avoiding adrenaline and ephedrine; using corticosteroids to maintain free breathing if necessary; and treating all acute attacks promptly.

୬

Women with epilepsy

Five women in every 1000 having a baby are subject to seizures. Though this is a small number, they have attracted hundreds of articles in the medical press. Few women have had the risks and benefits of continued treatment so fully examined because two known teratogens are used to treat epileptic women – phenytoin and sodium valproate (Valproic Acid). A third teratogen, trimethadione (troxidone), is no longer used. Epilepsy itself may be teratogenic and so women with epilepsy face very difficult decisions.

In most women the control of seizures is unchanged during pregnancy; some (17–37 per cent) experience an increase in seizures. For most women the risks of not taking medication, to herself and the fetus, are greater than the risk of continuing. During pregnancy the body uses up more of the anti-epileptic medication and dosages need to be monitored carefully. Some studies seem to show that seizures themselves carry risks. They note that a baby's heartbeat slows markedly during a seizure and remains low for as long as 20 minutes. Most babies would be able to cope with this but a few risk damage or even death from lack of oxygen, and stillbirths have been recorded. It appears that, very rarely, epilepsy seizures can cause a fall severe enough to damage the baby.

One study showed twice as many babies with a cleft palate born to mothers who experienced seizures but took no medication, than to mothers who had no seizures.

There is unanimity about the risk of some anti-epileptic drugs. Studies show that four times as many babies with cleft palate disorders are born to controlled epileptics, as to women who do not have the disease. There is an increased risk of heart malformations in babies. These are usually detectable on ultrasound scans well before the 16th week of pregnancy. It has also been found that neural tube defects, like spina bifida, occur in 1 per cent of women who take sodium valproate

(Valproic Acid) and, again, these may be seen on ultrasound around the sixteenth week of pregnancy.

As a general rule, about seven women in 100 who have epilepsy and take drugs to control it, have babies with congenital defects, about twice the rate found in the general population. If two or more anti-epileptic drugs are taken the risk increases to 15 per cent. The risk is also increased if larger doses are taken. Faced with this knowledge, some women just stop taking their medication. You may feel tempted to do the same but this is probably not the safest course to take. It would be better to sort out your choices with a doctor. This could be your own GP, though several epileptic women told me about how frustrating it was searching for doctors to ask their very specialized questions. A consultation with a neurologist might be one way. If this is not possible, voluntary groups for epileptics may help you sort out your options – you will find their address on page 256.

If you have been seizure-free for two years, then gradually withdrawing medication completely before your pregnancy is one option. It may also be possible to reduce it to the absolute minimum needed. The risks may be minimized by taking a single drug rather than a combination, unless this is necessary to control the epilepsy adequately. Switching from higher-risk drugs to carbamazepine is one approach to continued drug treatment, if it can be done, although there is still a risk of neural tube defects with carbamazepine, estimated to be 1 per cent in one study. Other studies have also implicated carbamazepine as a cause of birth defects.

Another reason to keep in close touch with your doctor is the need to monitor the changes in body chemistry that are the result of taking medication. This is especially important in pregnancy because some drugs can lower folate concentrations and decrease the amount of vitamins D and K available for you and your baby. By taking appropriate supplements you increase your baby's chances of being healthy. There is some evidence that taking folic acid supplements from before conception can reduce the risk of NTD, but this needs to be managed carefully because there is also evidence that high doses of folate can have a convulsant effect. Your baby will probably need supplements for a bit after he or she is born.

Most epileptics have normal babies. If you are taking medication, you still stand a good chance of being one of the 93 women in every 100 who do. I have met several. One said, 'Yes, do it! If I didn't have children, I would have felt abnormal but now I have five who are mine. They have asthma but aside from that, they're fine.' Another said:

I've taken phenytoin and primidone since I was a teenager. I did have genetic counselling before the first and heard about cleft palates and nice things like that. But I work in a paediatric unit so I know a cleft palate can be fixed. There were darker moments when I felt bleak and logic didn't work but mostly it did. I worried more about safety afterwards and did have a fit when Eve was three months old, but I woke to find I'd put her in her cot. I've never felt unsafe with them. I have three healthy children.

ॐ

Women who take minor tranquillizers

Benzodiazepine drugs – diazepam (Valium) and chlordiazepoxide (Librium) and a few others – are the most commonly-prescribed drugs in Western countries. It is estimated that 2 per cent of the British population takes the drug daily. Two out of three prescriptions are for women, many of whom will be of childbearing age and some of whom will become pregnant inadvertently or by design. Others may be pregnant yet continue to take the drug because they find the anxieties of pregnancy make the prospect of giving up too daunting. Some women may also take zodiazepine tranquillizers illegally, sometimes by injection. If you fit into any of these categories, you should ask for help from your doctor to gradually come off these tranquillizers, because that is the safest option for your baby. The risks associated with rapid withdrawal may well outweigh coming off it slowly, which involves taking a bit more of the drug.

What is the evidence about risk to the baby? Much of it is equivocal. One study suggested a slight rise in the number of babies with cleft palates (from one per thousand to 2 per thousand), but another looked at 611 infants with abnormal palates and found their mothers did not take benzodiazepines in large numbers and the authors concluded that something else caused the deformity. We do not really know whether these drugs are teratogenic in the first twelve weeks or what dosages may be harmful.

However, if you continue to take Valium* or Librium* in pregnancy, they will affect your baby. These drugs pass more easily into your baby than out again, and, over time, can accumulate. At birth, these babies are reluctant to breathe, slow to suck and find it hard to keep themselves warm. It takes patience and time to help these babies learn to breastfeed. Some babies may experience withdrawal symptoms and they will need careful observation. Sometimes, staff teach mothers what to look for; at others, these babies are cared for in the Special Care Baby Unit.

A one-off dose of benzodiazepines seems to have no ill effects. If you decide to do so, it is better to take single doses with ample time between for the baby to get rid of the drug. Your doctor will probably prescribe a version of the drug that is cleared more quickly from your system than Valium or Librium. Even so, there would need to be a pretty good reason to justify that decision. As the pressure groups who fight against the over-prescription of these drugs point out, minor tranquillizers don't touch the real cause of the problem nor help develop other ways of dealing with anxiety.

There is very little research available about neither drugs ('selective serotonin neuptake inhibitors') prescribed for depression such as fluoxetine (Prozac) and whether or not

---

* Neither is available on prescription in the UK under these trade names, only as diazepam and chlordiazepoxide respectively.

these are safe to use in pregnancy. Prozac does have side effects, like any drug, and these include nausea, vomiting and weight loss, which could adversely affect the baby.

One published study which looked at the effect of fluoxetine during early pregnancy concluded that it did not increase the risk of major malformations but, like tricyclic antidepressants, it may increase the risk of miscarriage. More research is needed before we can say whether or not Prozac is potentially teratogenic, and your doctor may recommend an alternative drug with a longer track record.

Voluntary groups such as TRANX have plenty of experience helping people stop taking drugs like Valium. Once you and your doctor have worked out a withdrawal plan, it could help to contact TRANX for support while you carry it out (address on page 256). That way, you and your baby will arrive at birth ready for life without these chemicals.

ॐ

Women taking lithium

One pregnant woman in a thousand takes lithium, most commonly to control manic depression. Lithium (sometimes called lithium carbonate) is a known teratogen. If a woman takes the drug in the first 12 weeks, there is five times more risk that her baby will have a heart defect. One study of 59 children born to women taking lithium found that nine were abnormal or died soon after birth, compared to one baby in 38 whose mothers had similar illnesses but were treated with other drugs.

If you take lithium and you are making a decision about having a baby, you need to decide whether to continue with it as it may damage your baby, or stop, thus risking a relapse which may also be harmful for you or your baby. Most women find this a difficult time and are grateful for all the help, support and nurturing others are willing to offer. One person who is sure to be involved is your doctor because pregnancy changes the way your body uses lithium, and, should you decide to continue to take it, the dosage will need to be adjusted.

This is not a decision that can be made quickly – most women take a long time to sort out the options. Withdrawal before pregnancy should be gradual – six to eight weeks seems to be the recommended time scale. It may take longer to work out new ways of coping with your illness before attempting pregnancy.

If you are taking lithium and discover you are unexpectedly pregnant, go and see your doctor immediately. He or she will probably suggest you stop taking the drug at once and substitute other less risky drugs to help you manage your illness. You will probably also be scheduled for an ultrasound investigation, as this often picks up cardiac abnormalities that might be present in your baby. There are voluntary groups who are experienced in supporting women who are unsure of their baby's health, or who are awaiting scans to gather more information. You will find addresses on page 256.

᭡

Women with diabetes

In contrast to some chronic illnesses such as epilepsy and manic depression, diabetes is more of a success story. Elevated blood sugar levels can increase the risk of complications, for example having a larger baby or a build up of fluid around the baby. But in the last few years, doctors have developed ways of monitoring blood sugar levels, adjusting insulin levels, and monitoring the baby's progress, so that well-controlled diabetic mothers can look forward to a pregnancy that lasts 40 weeks, and a baby that has almost the same chances as any other baby.

Good results are only possible if the woman and her medical team work smoothly together from well before pregnancy. This is very important because the chance of abnormal development in the first six weeks of pregnancy is still greater than the chance in non-diabetic women. How much greater is unclear – recent studies suggest it may be up to three times more likely. Where control is good, fewer babies are damaged. It also seems that 'hypos' (hypoglycaemic attacks) do not have any association with congenital abnormalities.

This is such a contrast from the way it used to be, and such a welcome change for diabetic women, most of whom are well aware of the importance of planning ahead (good news travels fast), that most do seek help before pregnancy. If you are thinking of having a baby, pregnancy will bring many changes – more regular testing at home, new insulin dosages, a different timetable for injections, new dietary restrictions, and more regular clinic visits. All these are worked out to suit your individual needs and most diabetic women seem to cope with new demands. Perhaps they, too, have caught the feeling of optimism and pride that doctors radiate when it comes to managing diabetes at this time.

The British Diabetic Association produces an information pack for diabetic women. It also runs a link scheme putting pregnant women in touch with experienced diabetic mothers so they can share feelings and experiences (see page 255).

Some women develop diabetes during pregnancy. Doctors call this gestational diabetes. The risk of minor elevation in blood sugar in pregnancy is unclear, and may not justify treatment, either through regulating diet or injectable insulin. However, between three and twelve women in every 100 may experience symptoms severe enough to require attention. Doctors no longer recommend pills to lower blood sugar (hypoglycaemic drugs), instead they prefer to treat the condition by limiting carbohydrates in the diet. Only if this doesn't work do they prescribe low doses of insulin for the rest of the pregnancy. This is so called 'gestational diabetes' usually disappears after the pregnancy. Some, but not all, of these women will develop diabetes in later life.

There is no evidence that insulin is harmful to babies. Untreated diabetes, however, can mean a 40 per cent mortality rate for babies. Those that survive may grow large enough to cause problems at delivery; they may have crises at birth due to abnormal blood sugar; and they may have problems with breathing due to immature lungs.

✥

Women with abnormal heart rhythms

The three drugs most commonly used to treat irregular heart beats are digoxin, quinidine and lignocaine.

Digoxin crosses the placenta and is only harmful if the mother's dose rises high enough to be too toxic for her own body. Then, the baby, too, receives too much of the drug. There are no reports of digoxin causing abnormalities in babies. A doctor will monitor the blood levels of digoxin regularly because pregnancy causes the mother's body to clear the drugs more rapidly.

There are no reports of quinidine causing birth defects or problems in pregnancy, if the dose stays within therapeutic limits. Again, doctors will monitor blood levels because pregnancy changes the way a woman's body uses the drug.

Lignocaine has also never been associated with teratogenesis, but information about this drug is sparse. It is usually used for short periods later in pregnancy. We are not sure how pregnancy changes the way a woman's body uses lignocaine.

✥

Women with high blood pressure

There are two types of high blood pressure (hypertension) which pregnant women might experience. One is a chronic problem and predates the pregnancy; the other is acute and is caused by the pregnancy itself, and is considered here in the 'chronic' section to make explaining easier.

Essential hypertension is a chronic problem. The blood pressure has been high for months or even years before the pregnancy, for reasons that have nothing to do with pregnancy. It is usually treated with methyldopa (Aldomet, Dopament, Hydromet, Medomet). This is the drug of choice because it has been used for a long time and reduces the risk of severe hypertension in women with moderate hypertension. Follow-up studies up to the age of seven show that children have no ill effects. But it has disadvantages, too. In 15 per cent of all cases, the side-effects are serious enough to make the drug intolerable. Many who take methyldopa are sleepy, depressed and prone to feeling faint when they stand up.

Women who cannot tolerate methyldopa may be offered beta blockers like propanolol, atenolol, metoprolol and labetalol and calcium channel blockers are increasingly being used. One doctor remarked, 'There is little to choose between the various beta blockers', though he noted that propanolol has been shown to slightly reduce the baby's growth in a tiny study of twelve babies. Beta blockers may have fewer side-effects then methyldopa but we don't have such a long follow-up on the babies and so we can be less confident that they are generally safe. Follow-up studies on women who took the drug show no higher rates of malformation than in the general population, but they are of such small numbers – 100 and 120 – that little can be made of their results.

The other kind of high blood pressure that can occur in pregnancy is called by many names including toxaemia, pre-eclampsia and pre-eclamptic toxaemia. It is usually said that the less people understand about something, the more names they give it, and this holds true here. Doctors call the symptom *pregnancy induced hypertension* or PIH, and continue to look for its underlying cause. We have no real idea why PIH happens.

Since doctors could not treat the cause, they tried for years to treat the symptoms, in the same way as they treated high blood pressure in non-pregnant people. One approach – giving methyldopa or hydrazaline as described above – has proved to be helpful and appears to be relatively safer, according to several small studies of women given the drug to lower PIH.

Beta-blockers, and more rarely diazoxide, have also been given to women with severe pregnancy-induced hypertension and pre-eclampsia. Like hydrazaline, labetalol and diazoxide cross the placenta. Labetalol may cause severe and long lasting brachycardia in the baby, especially after high doses. Diazoxide is not recommended because it is considered to have potential for harmful side effects – hyperglycaemia has been reported in some newborn babies whose mothers were given diazoxide. A recently published study which reviewed the literature on calcium channel blockers, suggest that the type II blockers such as nifedipine are safe for use in pregnancy.

The other approach was to lower blood pressure by giving thiazide diuretics like chlorothiazide, hydrochlorothiazide, or methylclothiazide. They work by lowering the amount of fluid circulating and thus reducing blood pressure and swelling caused by fluid retention. A review of trials conducted on women who took diuretics for PIH showed that no harm befell the babies, nor did the mothers have many side-effects, other than a few needing extra potassium. What the survey did not show was any difference in outcome between women with PIH who did take diuretics, and women who did not. The authors of the review concluded that, in view of the lack of benefit, diuretics are not worth the risk. As already noted earlier, calcium supplements and low dose aspirin have been proposed as possible ways to reduce the risk of PIH but there is not enough to justify taking either of these. Similarly there is not enough information to support reduced salt intake as a measure to reduce PIH.

Eclampsia can cause convulsions, a complication that occurs in one in 2,000 pregnancies in developed countries. Magnesium sulphate has been used for much of this century, although diazepam was introduced as an alternative in 1968, and phenytoin in 1987. A recent study by WHO in nine countries involving 1,680 women showed that magnesium sulphate was far more effective than the other two drugs, and also reduced the likelihood of women needing to be admitted

– their babies also fared better with magnesium sulphate. Another study also showed magnesium sulphate to be more effective than phenytoin in preventing eclamptic seizures. Diazepam only clears slowly from the baby's body, especially if given to the mother in high doses, causing problems with breathing and feeding.

There is no doubt that PIH can rise dangerously high, putting the mother and baby's life at risk in extreme cases. What is controversial is when to begin treating raised blood pressure, what degree of increase is worrying and what benefits may ensue for mother and baby. Each doctor will have his own regime and you will need to find out why and when your own begins treating PIH.

⟋⟍

Women taking anticoagulants

Anticoagulants (so-called 'blood thinners') are given to increase the amount of time it takes your blood to clot. They are used if the risk of a clot is high – after an artificial heart valve is put in, for instance, or following a clot in a vein. Between one and three women in every 1000 take anticoagulants in pregnancy. One doctor, after reviewing the options for treating them, concluded, 'Anticoagulant treatment should not be undertaken lightly in pregnancy. It poses additional risks to both the mother and the fetus. Further clinical trials are necessary to determine the best [management].'

Women who have artificial heart valves face the hardest choice. The drug that best keeps clots at bay is warfarin which is a known teratogen. It is thought that the risk that the baby will be damaged is about five in 100. However, one small study followed 22 women who took warfarin in the first 12 weeks and all produced normal babies. A variety of abnormalities have been associated with warfarin, including nasal defects, abnormal cartilage growth, central nervous system damage and bleeding into the baby's brain during labour.

Despite this some clinicians feel that if the woman has an artificial heart valve, warfarin remains the drug of choice for early pregnancy. They argue that the alternatives have not been studied or present even greater risks. Others disagree and recommend another drug – heparin – for the first 12 weeks, followed by warfarin after the period of maximum sensitivity has passed. This is a matter of clinical judgement and you will need to find out what your doctor recommends and the grounds for his or her belief.

After 36 weeks, most women switch to heparin, given by IV drip for two weeks, then stop it for 12 hours after which their labour is induced.

These can be very difficult decisions. One woman who had all the consequences explained when her new heart valve was put in four years earlier, said when she was 22 weeks pregnant:

> There's no other way for me to have a baby. It's this or nothing. I've had three scans to check out the baby and that seemed fine, so Pete and I are just crossing our fingers. We thought for months before trying for a baby and held our breaths for the first few months, because I know there is a high risk of miscarriage, but we made it this far. For me, I just say I've had trouble with my heart for years and life is still worth it so even if the baby has something, well we can cope with that.

Heparin is the other drug used to prevent clots forming in the mother's veins which could, if they break loose and travel to her lungs, cause her death. Doctors recommend that a woman should begin the drug in pregnancy if a clot forms because, on balance, that seems safest. They are less keen to prescribe heparin if a woman simply has a history of clots in the past. Another alternative to drugs is to teach her the symptoms to look out for and recommend she gets in touch should any occur. You will need to discuss the pros and cons of taking heparin to keep clots at bay.

Heparin is one of the rare examples of a drug that only crosses the placenta in minute amounts (if at all) because its molecules are enormous compared to those of other drugs. Theoretically, then, it poses no risk to the baby. But it may have dangerous side effects that put the mother at risk. One problem is loss of minerals from her bones (osteoporosis); in one study of twenty women, one developed osteoporosis and in another study 30 per cent of a small group of pregnant women taking heparin were found to have suffered reduced bone density. She is also at risk of bleeding when taking heparin. The drug can be hard to administer because a woman either has to remain in hospital for the injections or she has to learn to give them to herself. Frequent lab tests to check the dosage and effect are also needed.

჻

Women with hyperthyroidism

Three drugs are used to treat over-activity of the thyroid gland – carbimazole, propylthiouracil and methimazole. If your thyroid is overactive, it is safer for your baby if you treat the condition, as hyperthyroidism can cause abnormal development in the baby and premature labour. Carbimazole is said to be the drug of choice.

There is no evidence that these drugs directly change how your baby develops, however, because carbimazole crosses the placenta, it will make a difference to how your baby's thyroid gland functions, just as it does your own. Excessive dosages can result in hypothyroidism (too little of the hormone) and occasionally goitre in the baby. The dose should be carefully monitored via monthly blood tests to measure free thyroxine and thyroid stimulating hormone; and it is recommended that carbimazole is stopped at 37 weeks and recommended after birth. Propylthiouracil may be a better alternative to carbimazole because it does not cross the placenta so readily, but it is also believed to affect the baby's thyroid gland. All babies will need careful monitoring when they are born to make sure they can readjust to life without anti-hyperthyroid drugs.

Some women have hypothyroidism, and their pre-pregnancy dose of thyroxine may need to be increased during pregnancy, because the dosage is weight-related. However there appears to be no danger to the baby – in fact it is more dangerous to stop treatment because this increases the risk of miscarriage, premature labour and abnormality.

Women with Herpes

Herpes simplex virus can be transmitted to the baby with devastating effects including miscarriage, early labour, poor growth and neurological problems. Fortunately, this happens in only two in every 100,000 pregnancies in the UK. Less fortunately treatment is less clear. Acyclovir has been tried in pregnancy and does not seem to increase the risk of congenital defects. Larger trials are underway and we need to wait for results of these before it will be possible to say whether acyclovir is beneficial and to assess potential risks to the baby.

Women with HIV

If you have HIV you may be receiving treatment for the virus itself or for the opportunistic infections which are more common in people with HIV (because their immune systems are affected by the virus). You will need to weigh up with your doctor the risks and benefits of drug treatment for different infections.

How safe is zidovudine (AZT), the antiretroviral drug given to people with HIV, during pregnancy? A (1994) important trial reported that when pregnant women with HIV (but who were not seriously ill) were given zidovudine from 14 weeks onwards, transmission of the virus to the baby was dramatically reduced. (We know that HIV can be transmitted to the baby from the mother – studies have suggested that the risk is about one in five.) The study concluded that HIV positive pregnant women should be given zidovudine for their own benefit as well as that of their babies.

Studies in animals and small trials of the drug in pregnant women have so far shown no association with abnormalities, although the women in the American study mentioned were not given the drug until after 14 weeks gestation so we cannot judge possible teratogenicity in the first trimester. The Antiretroviral Pregnancy Register, which is maintained by the manufacturers of zidovudine with the US Centers for Disease Control, has found no evidence of an increased risk of congenital abnormalities in babies of 121 women given the drug during pregnancy.

On the basis of what we know, the benefits of ziduvodine outweigh any potential risks of use during pregnancy. However, we do not know very much yet about the long term effects on the baby of zidovudine treatment in pregnancy.

ॐ

In conclusion

Nearly every chronic illness has a voluntary support group that is often the best source of up-to-date information and support. Many are beginning to take the particular needs of pregnant women into account, publishing special information sheets or setting up link-schemes. And others would do so if they were asked for this kind of advice more often. Many women I spoke to when investigating these issues said that talking to other women who have had similar experiences was the most helpful thing. You, too, might have similar luck if you contact the appropriate support group. If they do not know the answer, being asked might spur them to find out.

❧ 10 ❧

Over-the-Counter and Kitchen Drugs in Pregnancy

This chapter is about substances you might not consider drugs at all, at first glance. You can buy them over the counter at the chemist's or you can find them in your kitchen cupboard. You could consider them so much a part of your life that they do not seem worth thinking about. But they are drugs.

So what is a 'drug'? Any chemical that gets into your bloodstream and changes the way your body works could be considered a 'drug'. By this criteria, the caffeine in your coffee, the fluoride in the water, the wine you drank last night and the headache tablets you took this morning, are all drugs. It is worth thinking about each of them in terms of their consequences for you and, once you are pregnant, for your developing baby.

I have known women to get carried away with the notion that everything has to be re-evaluated – it can definitely be taken too far. If you cast a net wide enough to encompass all you eat, drink or inhale, you will feel surrounded by dangers. At the very least, it could make you feel very anxious; but it is more likely that you would be paralysed by too many choices. It is not your responsibility to investigate all of the possible chemicals around you and you couldn't, even if it was a good idea, because *everything* carries a potential risk. A 1983 paper on risk assessment reminded the over-wary that, 'If sugar and salt were considered as food additives and subjected to studies as to their acute toxicity, lifetime effects, carcinogenicity, reproductive toxicity, and genetic toxicity ... neither would be permitted for use in food.'

So, after acknowledging how wide an investigation into freely available drugs in pregnancy *might* go, it seems useful to pull back and examine the ones that are known to affect a developing baby. This chapter will review what the journals are talking about and what the women themselves ask about when they are given the chance. It will not cover alcohol, tobacco and illegal or street drugs, as each deserves a chapter on its own.

ᗡ

A pill for every ill?

People spend billions on over-the-counter medications. The most common drugs available without prescription and taken by pregnant women are, pain-relieving drugs, like aspirin and paracetamol, cough and cold remedies, drugs to relieve digestive problems, vitamins and drugs to relieve skin and muscle problems.

It is now much less common for pregnant women to report taking over-the-counter medications than it used to be. A 1986 study repeated a survey done in 1971 that found 65 per cent of women took non-prescription drugs; 15 years later, only 9 per cent said they did. Other studies have found the figures higher than this one but all note a downward trend. One doctor notes the cause as the '... continued attention paid by the news media to drug induced fetal abnormality'.

He is probably right. Ask any pregnant woman and she will probably reply. 'I just don't take anything.' Not all will include drugs like aspirin in such statements.

In fact, year by year, the general population consumes *more* over-the-counter medications than in the past. Most people consider it odd to put up with a discomfort when a pharmaceutical remedy is at hand. If you have a headache, take an aspirin. Tummy upset? Manufacturers spend millions convincing us to reach for this tablet or that liquid. Feeling anxious? Not to worry – there's a pill to calm you. All life's ups and down need pharmaceutical solutions if the advertisers are to be believed.

Pregnant women grow up with these attitudes and then they are suddenly expected to live by new rules – it becomes 'No pills regardless of the ills and just put up with the discomfort'. Ironically, for many women, pregnancy is the first time they feel the need for any pills and potions. It is often the first time in their lives that they feel truly awful. Doctors may refer to their symptoms as 'the minor discomforts of pregnancy' but for the women concerned, there's nothing 'minor' about feeling sick, tired, achey or in pain – sometimes all at once: 'For the first few weeks it was like I was hung over and I couldn't do anything about it. I just lived from one day to another.'

Most women find that they put up with the 'minor discomforts' and many find non-pharmaceutical ways to help themselves feel better. Any general pregnancy book will suggest ways to ease discomforts and other pregnant women will tell you what helped them. For example, some women find osteopathy can help to alleviate the symptoms of sciatica back pain, and carpal tunnel syndrome, which many experience during pregnancy. But osteopathy should be avoided if there is any history of or threatened miscarriage, and is usually avoided around the twelfth and sixteenth weeks when miscarriage is more likely to occur. Many of these suggestions are better than drugs because they get to the root of the problem, rather than just treating the symptoms. A non-pharmaceutical remedy is not a 'second best' remedy, but it may take a while to get used to thinking this way.

But there may be times when you consider over-the-counter drugs to alleviate symptoms or to help should you become ill. The following information may help you weigh up the risks and benefits of such a decision.

ॐ

Aspirin

One study found that 45 per cent of all pregnant women take aspirin at some time in their pregnancy. Many take it in the early weeks before they know they are pregnant, and then they worry about the effects on the baby. The evidence we have about aspirin comes from many different sources. In animals, when given in very large doses, aspirin does increase the number of offspring who are malformed. This suggests there may be some link between aspirin and malformation and most doctors recommend avoiding aspirin in the first trimester of pregnancy to be on the safe side. However, huge studies in humans have failed to show any link. One study of 50,000 women found no more abnormalities in the babies of women who took aspirin compared to those who did not. Another study of 14,000 confirmed that finding. Indeed, studies have been done to see if daily doses of aspirin of one-tenth of the normal dose, given after the fourteenth week of pregnancy, will decrease the incident of high blood pressure and help babies at risk of growing poorly to reach a more normal size. The early results are promising, although larger studies are needed before this treatment becomes standard practice. But the willingness of ethics committees to contemplate such trials point to the conclusion that aspirin is probably not terato-genic, at least after the first trimester.

This does not mean that aspirin has no effect on the baby, because aspirin acts on many different systems in the body. When anyone takes aspirin – either directly by mouth or via the placenta – that person will make less of a hormone called prostaglandin. For the baby before birth, prostaglandins are involved in keeping open a blood vessel that allows the baby's blood to by-pass the lungs (clearly useful as the baby does not breathe before it is born). Less prostaglandin means a higher risk that the baby's lung 'by-pass' will close too early. This is not a risk with a one-off dose now and again, but 13 per cent of women in one study report taking aspirin several times a week, usually for headaches. In view of this complication, these women are advised to seek other ways of alleviating the problem.

Another effect is a change in how your blood clots. Anyone who takes aspirin will have blood that clots more slowly because one component of clotting, the platelets, do not stick together as well. This effect lasts for up to five days after taking the drug and makes you and the baby more prone to bleeding during that time. Some studies suggest that tiny bleeds may upset the baby's normal development if the mother takes repeated full doses of aspirin (eight or more times a week, in one study). While the odd aspirin occasionally may not do any harm, if you find yourself taking more than the occasional dose in pregnancy, you need to explore with your doctor other ways of treating whatever is wrong.

High doses may increase the risk of material or newborn bleeding, and it would also be wise to avoid aspirin towards the end of the pregnancy to make sure you and your baby are not more prone to bleeding during the birth. Taking aspirin near birth may also increase the chance that your baby will be jaundiced.

⁓

Acetaminophen/Paracetamol

We know much less about the effect of paracetamol on the baby than we do about aspirin. It does cause abnormalities in rats but no one has documented any teratogenic effects in humans. Unlike aspirin, it does not increase the risk of bleeding or have a lasting effect on the amount of prostaglandins available to the baby. For this reason, many doctors recommend it for use in pregnancy.

Others, however, disagree. They say that the reason it seems generally safe is that there have not been many tests of the effects. It's true that we know more about the adverse effects of aspirin but that is because we know more about aspirin in general. These doctors argue that we are perhaps safer with the 'bad news' we know, than optimistically hoping that no news is good news. And because we do not know enough about their safety, other pain killers such as ibuprofen should generally be avoided.

One thing both camps agree on is that either aspirin or paracetamol *should* be used if you have a fever. On balance, the small risks associated with these medications are outweighed by the risks to the baby of a high temperature. Earlier studies linked fever in the mother in the first three months of pregnancy, with malformation, but this now seems unlikely. However, other problems like prematurity and stillbirth are more likely if the core temperature (the temperature inside a mother's body) rises too high. That's why women are advised to take aspirin or paracetamol to bring fever down, to avoid hot baths or saunas when feverish, and to wear light clothing.

৵

Cold remedies

No drug can cure a cold but some claim to alleviate the symptoms. As there are dozens of variations and brand names to choose from, the only way to know what is in the medication you are thinking of taking, is to read the label. When you do, you will find as many as seven drugs combined in one remedy. They will probably include:

- *aspirin or paracetamol* – Either is useful in helping you feel better but it is cheaper and more accurate to take it separately. This way, you know how much you are taking – an important point in view of the adverse effects described above.
- *something to dry up secretions* – These are usually given in such small doses that they have no effect or, if they do, they may even prolong the infection by interfering with the body's ability to fight it off. Used as a nasal spray, decongestants

cause a 'rebound' effect – they do dry out the lining of your nose but when the effect wears off, your nose will be even runnier than before. Some decongestants (ephedrine, phenyl-propanolamine, phenyephrine) have been associated with birth defects in a study of 50,000 women, but the level is not statistically significant and the defects could have been caused by the virus, not the medication. However, none are worth the risk because they offer no benefit for the mother.

- *a stimulant* – Usually caffeine (see page 119).

Combining several drugs in a fixed ratio means it is very unlikely that you will receive the correct dose of any one of them, and taking a time-release capsule means it is very unlikely that you will ever have enough of the drug to do any good. Taking a proprietary cold remedy when you are pregnant makes no sense, and not much more sense when you are not.

Some cold remedies also contain antihistamines, but there is no real evidence that they do any good.

$\backsim$

Cough medicines

Cough medicines, like cold remedies, come in dozens of different forms.

- Some are sold as *expectorants* with ingredients like potassium iodide, ammonium chloride, sodium citrate, ipecacuanha, creosote, eucalyptus, menthol and benzoin compounds. These have never been shown to be effective and one expert calls the claims about expectorants 'expensive myths'.
- Some are sold as *lozenges* you suck to suppress a cough. None has been shown to be any more effective than sucking an ordinary sweet. Codeine does suppress a cough if used in large enough doses, however pregnant women should avoid it as it has been linked with birth defects, and it will cause dependency in the baby if it is used regularly.

- Most are *combinations* and it is difficult to know what drugs they contain.

Some drugs sold as cough remedies have proved no more effective at alleviating symptoms than sugar solutions. These include: Dimeotapp, Actifed and Benylin. Cough medicines containing iodides should probably be avoided. Iodides can cross the placenta and in larger doses can potentially harm the baby – they have been linked with goitre (enlargement of the thyroid gland) and hyperthyroidism (overactivity of the thyroid gland).

Most cough medications are useless, some are harmful and most are expensive. There is no benefit to balance against even a tiny risk to your baby, and, if you are pregnant, your best bet is to suck something to soothe your throat, drink plenty of warm liquids, use a steam inhaler if you have one and wait for the cough to pass. If it doesn't, go and see your doctor.

࿓

Drugs for heartburn and digestive problems

Most pregnant women find heartburn a problem in the last two or three months of pregnancy. By then, your baby is big enough to push upward on your stomach from below. At the same time, the ring of muscle that normally keeps the acidic stomach contents from entering the oesophagus has relaxed due to hormone changes in pregnancy, so the stomach contents slosh upwards and you feel a burning pain just under your breastbone.

You can ease the pain by eating frequent small meals, taking enough to eat avoiding acid, spicy foods, sleeping with several pillows and not bending over. If possible it is better to avoid antacids and to have a milky drink instead. However, if heartburn is getting you down, a chemical that neutralizes the acid in your oesophagus will probably help. Doctors recommend that you take something that will not pass out of the stomach into your bloodstream because that way little will reach the baby. After 12 weeks, most of the baby's organs are formed anyway and they are less vulnerable to harm.

The best way to get hold of an antacid is to talk to your doctor or midwife. They will have some standard remedy for pregnant women. However, if you are in need and you cannot wait for your next appointment, you can get antacids without prescription. If you find yourself standing in front of a shelf full of brand names, here are some guidelines:

• Read all the labels carefully and don't choose anything that does not detail its contents
• Don't use sodium bicarbonate because it is absorbed from the stomach and changes your body chemistry
• Magnesium carbonate is also absorbed into the bloodstream
• Avoid any antacid containing bismuth because no one knows its effect on the baby
• Antacids based solely on aluminium salts are not recommended because they interfere with the absorption of iron and they are very constipating
• Antacids are based on mixtures of bases containing aluminium, magnesium and calcium seem to work best
• Tablets which can be sucked bring more relief because they reach the oesophagus in small doses.

The next time you see your midwife or doctor, you can discuss the matter with them. (Remember, antacids are only used fairly freely in the last third of pregnancy; babies whose mothers took antacids in early pregnancy have slightly higher rates of abnormality than those whose mothers did not.)

Other remedies such as prostigmine have been shown to help with no apparent hazard from occasional use, but the safety of guinetidine or omeprozole has not been established for use in pregnancy.

ॐ

Constipation in pregnancy

Constipation troubles many pregnant women. Some find it a problem from the moment they know they are pregnant; others are only bothered towards the end of pregnancy as the growing baby presses on the intestinal tract. Hormones, too, make the gut muscle less efficient at moving its contents along.

Treatment for constipation lies in helping your body work more efficiently by adding bulk to your diet and ensuring you drink plenty of fluid. Increase the amount of bran you eat, choose fresh fruit and vegetables and whole grains, and drink plenty of fluids, then you will probably find that you are not overly troubled by constipation. If these measures are not enough, you could try a bulk-forming laxative such as lactu-lose solution BP (lactulose) or ispaghula husk (fybogen). These contain substances like gum, agar, cellulose or methyl-cellulose which absorb water, keeping the contents of your intestines soft. They all require you to drink plenty of fluids in order to work properly. Because they stay in the intestines and do not reach your baby, they are considered to be safe.

Some laxatives are designed to soften the stool and lessen the need for straining. This may be helpful for some women but you need to be careful which preparation you choose. Your doctor or midwife will be used to advising women on which is best. Mineral oils such as liquid paraffin should be avoided as they interfere with the absorption of many fat soluable vita-mins and minerals, including vitamin K which is an essential part of blood clotting. Liquid paraffin is absorbed from the gut and can cause side-effects.

Some laxatives are based on chemicals that irritate the lining of the large intestine, stimulating it to contract quickly and empty. Dozens of brands are available. The chemicals used include bisacodyl, phenolphthalein, alse, senna, cascara, castor oil, fig, sodium picosulphate and danthron. Some are taken by mouth, others are suppositories. They can cause cramping and excess fluid loss, and chronic use may disturb the normal functioning of the bowels. They may also cross the placenta and we know little about their possible effects on the baby. They should therefore be used with caution at all times but especially towards the end of pregnancy, as the strong contractions caused by some preparations (for example, castor oil) may precipitate labour. Some women have, in the past, used castor oil for just this end, but many women find the rather violent diarrhoea uncomfortable when it coincides with contractions.

Salts of magnesium, sodium, and potassium, in various combinations (for example Milk of Magnesia, Andrews Liver Salts, Epsom Salts), should be avoided as they are absorbed in large enough amounts to cause problems for the baby's kidneys. The only way to tell if a laxative contains these salts is to read the label. If any of these three elements – sodium, potassium, or magnesium – form part of the chemical named, avoid the preparation.

The best course is to change your diet to accommodate the new demands of pregnancy. One woman said (albeit with a rueful smile):

I never knew there were so many ways to use bran ... bran scones, bran muesli, bran in casseroles, bran bread! Even Ian began to 'think brown' when I was pregnant.

ॐ

Leg Cramps

Some women suffer from leg cramps during pregnancy. A range of things have been claimed to help – from quinine henadryl, vitamin D, to calcium supplements, but there is no evidence from any studies to support these claims.

᠈ᢣᢣ

Vitamins in pregnancy

See Chapter 7.

᠈ᢣᢣ

Skin disorders in pregnancy

You should be careful about considering drugs to apply to your skin. Even if the skin is not broken the drug will be absorbed to a greater or lesser extent and once it is in your body, it will reach your baby, too. This applies equally to drugs taken for skin disorders. As mentioned earlier, isotretinoin, a drug used to treat acne, was found to be highly teratogenic.

Aches and sore muscles are best treated with a warm bath and friendly massage. Skin problems can often be cured in the same way. If you choose to use a cream or lotion on your skin, be especially wary of:

- *antibiotic creams* – Some contain tetracycline and any could sensitize a baby allergic to that particular antibiotic.
- *anti-itching medications* – These may contain antihistamines and corticosteroids which are useful when used on a small area, but they are not suitable for the general itching many pregnant women feel as they then need to be applied to a large area. A soothing bath may be better or, in desperation, a lotion such as calamine lotion, which is relatively inert. Corticosteroids carried no increased risk to the baby when taken for asthma (see page 89).
- *antifungal preparations* – Thrush is very common in pregnancy and you should report any vaginal discharge that is itchy or foul smelling. Topical imidazoles (which are more effective than nystatin) applied to the affected area may be prescribed (see page 81).

- *anti-parasitic preparations* – These are used to treat scabies and lice infestations and up to 10 per cent of the applied drug is absorbed into the body. Lindane is found in some preparations to treat the problem and it should be avoided; we know of one case of severe birth defects in a mother who used it in the first third of pregnancy. Carbaryl and malathion are both effective and neither has been reported as causing problems for the baby.
- *vaginal deodorants* – These have no place in pregnancy as many contain hexachlorophane, a drug linked with birth defects in animals. Any drug will be absorbed more easily by the mucous membranes around the vagina than elsewhere on the body.

꒰

Kitchen drugs in pregnancy

It may not occur to you that your kitchen cupboards, as well as your bathroom medicine chest, may hold substances that need a re-think once you are pregnant. Alcohol is one drug you need to consider carefully and Chapter 12 considers this in detail. Others are less well known. For example, one pregnant woman was admitted to an emergency room complaining of heart palpitations, blurred vision and feeling very agitated. It turned out that she had eaten some homemade biscuits made with one tablespoon of nutmeg instead of the recommended teaspoon. Her baby was fine when he was born, and she was too, after 24 hours of treatment.

Other women turn to their spice shelf for help in pregnancy. Some now recommend ginger for morning sickness. Take as ginger biscuits or ginger tea (a spoonful or two steeped in boiling water and with lemon or honey to taste) or in capsules bought in a health food shop, or chewed in candied form, it does help some women to feel better. One enthusiastic grandmother, describing her daughter's misery through two pregnancies before trying ginger, wrote, 'It worked beautifully.'

ૐ

Caffeine

Caffeine is an 'everyday' drug found in coffee, tea, some fizzy drinks such as colas, chocolate, and several pain-relieving tablets from the chemist. It acts as a mild stimulant and most of us have some every day for just this effect. However, too much caffeine – say ten cups of coffee a day – makes most people feel anxious or restless, they have trouble going to sleep and they complain of headaches and heart palpitations. One Canadian study found that women who drank a lot of coffee – more than ten cups a day – had a slightly increased risk of miscarriage, premature birth and congenital heart defects, and animal studies have shown an association between caffeine and fetal loss. But another study published in 1993 showed no increased risk in women who consumed 300 mg caffeine/day – or three cups of filter coffee, three to four cups of instant coffee or tea, or five to six cans of cola. One problem with these studies is that caffeine consumption varies during pregnancy, and cup sizes and caffeine content of drinks made by different women also vary. So drawing conclusions is difficult.

In pregnancy, most doctors recommend that you stay below three 'servings' a day because it takes three times as long for your body to get rid of caffeine in pregnancy as when you are not pregnant. This probably makes sense on the basis of what we can glean from available research – excessive caffeine may be harmful, but three 'servings' a day does not appear to pose a risk.

But the caffeine you consume does reach your baby, causing him or her to experience the same mild stimulant effect as you do. As long as it is in your blood (and in pregnancy, that's a long time), caffeine tightens your blood vessels and reduces blood flow to the placenta. This is not a good thing for any growing baby, but it is especially worrying if you smoke. There is a good deal of evidence that suggests that caffeine increases the harmful effects of tobacco on the fetus.

This probably happens because smokers usually have larger placentas than non-smokers (see page 149). A bigger placenta is probably the body's way of trying to compensate for the chemicals in tobacco that make the placenta less efficient. Women who consume large amounts of caffeine (10 'servings' a day) and smoke 15 cigarettes a day, do not show the same increase in placenta size as women who smoke fifteen cigarettes and avoid caffeine. Apparently, caffeine keeps the blood-flow to the smaller placenta lower than it should be and interferes with its growth. The baby nourished by this placenta is already stunted by smoking and then further compromised by the effects of caffeine.

Many pregnant women now avoid caffeine entirely because they don't want to worry about even a small risk. It also helps them feel they are doing something positive for their babies and themselves. Others cut down on the caffeine they consume in a day and that, too, makes good sense in light of the facts given above. A few may worry that they might have harmed the baby by continuing to drink tea and coffee before they knew they were pregnant. They will be reassured to hear that there is very little evidence that exists to support this view. All women should look at the amount of caffeine they consume and judge if they, and their babies, would benefit from consuming less.

~

Wariness as a part of life

Taking care does not have to be a burden. Before a baby is born, parents spend time 'nesting' as they prepare the baby's room and organize clothes and cots. They could do the same sort of 'nesting' at the beginning of pregnancy by going through their medicine chest and throwing away anything that is left over, anything they no longer know the contents of and anything they know could be harmful to the baby. Then ask your doctor about what's left and consider carefully any drug you decide to take from the time you stop using contraceptives to the time your baby is weaned. During that time, you and your baby will be taking the drug together.

⁊ 11 ⁊

Herbal, and Homeopathic and Other Remedies in Pregnancy

You could be one of the many women who have used alternative medicines such as herbs or homeopathy for years and wish to carry on once you are pregnant. Or you could become interested in what seems a gentler, more natural approach to minor illnesses once a growing baby is part of the decision. You may know lots of women who use both herbs and homeopathic medicines in pregnancy. I suspect the number is growing as what was once seen as fringe medicine gains recognition by doctors and the general public.

Although these remedies are outside the boundaries of mainstream medicine, they still need to conform to the criteria you would apply to any other drug in pregnancy. Before you reach for the herbal tea, or accept someone else's arnica pills for your backache, you should ask yourself:

- Is it effective? If a remedy helps you or your baby, some extra risk may be worthwhile. If it offers no benefit, taking it makes no sense even if the risk is minute.
- Is it safe? Anything you do has risks but you need to assess whether the risks of using these remedies are small enough, or the benefits great enough, to justify it. As with any drug, what is safe for you and what is safe for your growing baby may be two very different things.

৵

Herbs in pregnancy

The benefits of herbal remedies

Herbs have wide-ranging benefits, many of which have nothing to do with their pharmaceutical properties. Anne McIntyre in her book, *Herbs for Pregnancy and Childbirth*, calls herbs 'the medicine of the people': by collecting, using and choosing herbs, a woman reclaims her independence from medical doctors who so often use pregnancy as an illness that they alone can 'cure'. Herbalists remind us that people are more than a collection of molecules because each one of us shares in the 'vital force' that keeps us well and maintains the body's systems in balance. If one views the world this way, disease becomes the by-product of disharmony and imbalance. Plants in their natural state, are seen as one way of eliminating disharmony and strengthening the body's own healing power. Using herbs is consistent with this world view. Herbs also link the user to others following similar dictums over many generations. Self-help, a sense of connection with other users, and help with particular problems can make women feel more in control and more confident about their bodies.

There are other less fundamental benefits. Herbs often smell lovely; they are relatively cheap; and they help us feel connected to the Earth and growing things, a need that can be especially strong in pregnancy.

The pharmacological benefits of herbs are harder to assess. Books abound about herbs, all describing the benefit and balm they have brought for specific problems. However, it is difficult to evaluate these claims because, as Anne McIntyre admits, 'there have yet been no studies carried out in maternity wards or antenatal clinics and hence no scientific assessments of the use of herbal medicine in modern maternity care'. Some animal tests have been done but the results are equivocal. Squaw vine, a remedy often suggested for pregnant women, based on the experience of American Indians, has no effect on guinea pigs. Arnica does enhance wound healing in animals. Drawing conclusions for humans only from animal studies is bad medicine.

So, in answer to the question, 'Do herbs work?' you have only the testimony of other women who say they do such as those who find that camomile tea or peppermint tea helps to alleviate morning sickness, and others who have said:

I drank gallons of raspberry leaf tea through this pregnancy and I didn't get so tired as in my former one. My labour was short and easy.

Cramp bark is a wonderful remedy for any kind of tension and restlessness in pregnancy.

Squaw vine and raspberry leaf together meant I had a much shorter labour this time. I started using them about six weeks before Willow was born and felt strong and ready for labour when it happened.

Each woman will make up her own mind about such testimony and consider her own experience before deciding whether or not to use herbs.

The risks of herbal remedies

Because herbs are sold as natural products, packaged to look like medicines, and sold in health food shops, the fantasy has grown that herbs are utterly safe. Not so. Wild herbs can be contaminated with pesticides or they can be mislabelled. Exceeding the recommended dose can lead to adverse effects while controlling the dose can be tricky given that different herbs, gathered at different times and prepared in different ways, will vary in strength. Though many advocates stress the naturalness of herbs ('Herbs are grown from the earth and contain the elements of the earth just as our physical bodies do'), many natural things are deadly poisonous as anyone who munched their way through their own garden would quickly discover. Nor is traditional wisdom and long experience any guarantee of safety. A few herbs that were once widely used are now to be avoided:

- comfrey – this can cause liver cancer and liver damage
- berberis – this is toxic to the liver
- ragwort – also toxic to the liver
- prickly ash – stomach problems, blood disorders
- apricot/plum/peach/pear/cherry seeds – cyanide poisoning
- ginseng – vaginal bleeding, swollen painful breasts (if used in excess) and should not be taken in conjunction with caffeine or where there is a history of hypertension or headaches
- feverfew – ulceration of mouth and tongue

Using any herb requires knowledge and caution, but this is even more true in pregnancy. All the books say a pregnant woman should not treat herself with herbs. Herbals teas sold for their flavour and comfort (such as camomile, cinnamon and others) are not a problem. If you are watching your daily caffeine intake, you may want to read the packet carefully as some teas contain as much as half the amount found in coffee.

Herbs sold as remedies are another matter. If the packet does not say what they contain, you have no idea what you are taking. Some herbs are known to be risky for pregnant women and their babies, for example aloe vera is linked with birth defects. The herbs listed below cause uterine contractions and have been linked with miscarriage.* The recommendation is that these herbs be avoided completely in the first six months of pregnancy, and then taken only cautiously after that. A few are suggested once labour has begun. Whereas ginger for example, which stimulates local circulation, should be avoided when birth is imminent.

---

* This list in one of the longest I have ever encountered but other authors produce slightly different lists.

arbor vitae	male fern
autumn crocus	mistletoe
barberry	mugwort
blue cohosh	nutmeg
broom	pennyroyal
cotton root	poke root
feverfew	rue
golden seal	southern wood
greater celandine	tansy
juniper	thuja
life root	wormwood

From Herbs for Pregnancy and Childbirth by Anne McIntyre (Sheldon, 1988)

Other authors have also suggested that the following herbs should also be avoided during pregnancy: lethroot, black cohosh, bryony cinchona, marjoram, meadow saffron, motherwort, safe and squaw vine.

The medical literature on the subject records individual cases where herbs have led to tragedy. A woman bought a herbal tea from a Swiss pharmacy which claimed to be an expectorant (it made it easier to cough up phlegm) and drank a cup a day throughout her pregnancy. Her baby died soon after birth from a fatal liver abnormality caused by the toxic build-up of alkaloids present in the tea. A survey of traditional herbal remedies in East Africa found much the same problem on a wide scale. About 20 per cent of the children treated for malnutrition failed to respond to intravenous therapy and supplemental feeding. The author concluded that these children had been given traditional herbal remedies either after birth or via their mothers during pregnancy, that resulted in damage to the liver.

Another study in South Africa found that herbal teas used for general wellbeing in pregnancy and as a treatment for constipation made the babies much more likely to empty their bowels, too. This is usually seen as a sign of lack of oxygen during labour and caregivers could misjudge this sign, seeing problems when none were present, or ignore real difficulties. The babies are also at increased risk of inhaling bowel contents at birth leading to a dangerous form of pneumonia.

This is not to say that all herbs are dangerous. There is no evidence of danger for most herbs when used in the prescribed amounts. To use them as safely as possible, you could consult the publications listed as references for this Chapter and you will need the guidance of a herbal practitioner who is well trained, experienced and interested in pregnancy. Anyone can call himself or herself a herbalist: some will be self-taught; many will have only a brief correspondence training; some will have trained for several years. Any reputable practitioner will welcome queries about his or her training and experience.

The organizations listed on page 255 are only some of the many umbrella organizations who publish directories of practitioners but inclusion does not necessarily signify competence. The consumer dictum 'Let the buyer beware ...' applies. If you do find a good herbalist, you are likely to get the kind of personal, caring, individual attention that the mainstream doctors often find hard to match – so the search is probably worth the effort, if you decide herbs are for you.

ↄ⸚

Homeopathy in pregnancy

The benefits of homeopathy

Homeopathy dates from about 1800 when a German physician, Samuel Hahnemann, announced that giving someone who was ill substances which would produce similar symptoms in healthy people actually helped. These substances, derived from plants, animals or minerals, were often poisonous when used in concentrated amounts, but in homeopathic doses, they were diluted again and again according to strict rules, then, it is claimed, in some way becoming more powerful in the process. This is called 'the magic of the minimal dose'.

In the intervening centuries, homeopathy has evolved an extensive body of literature describing how, when and in what amounts various homeopathic remedies should be prescribed. All the books I consulted agree that pregnancy is a particularly appropriate time for using homeopathy. They describe specific remedies for most of the minor ailments and for psychological upsets such as stress, fear and anxiety as well as for example Ipechacuanha for morning sickness. However, their bibliographies refer only to the original eighteenth century work or cite other books who in turn, refer to Hahnemann's work.

A wider search of the literature produced a few animal studies that show that homeopathic remedies have an effect that is slightly greater than the placebo effect but the evidence is very scarce. All the medical articles and references published in the world are collected in a database in Switzerland. I searched the database to corroborate the claims which are relevant to pregnancy, asking, as one always does at the beginning of such an exercise, for all articles on a particular topic – in this case, pregnancy and labour. There were over 900 articles. I then asked for articles in English about homeopathy and pregnancy. There were four, and three were, like books on homeopathy, articles *describing* homeopathic treatments used in midwifery and asserting their usefulness. The fourth was a case history of an individual woman's experience. As far as I can tell, there is no research data as to the effectiveness of homeopathy in pregnancy. Arnica, cansophyllum, chamomilla and pulsatilla are most commonly mentioned homeopathic preparations for birth (for more information see Complimentary Therapies in Pregnancy and Childbearing) and there are plenty of women who are convinced that homeopathy helped them:

I took Arnica this time and three days after Emily was born, my perineum was completely fine. No soreness or bruising. After Harry, it took weeks to feel better.

I swear by Nux Vomica 6X for morning sickness. I felt sick all day long before I took it, then only bad in the mornings when I did.

I was overdue with Joshua and determined not to have an induction this time, so I took Caulophyllum 6c and two days later I was in labour. It worked for me.

You may also have experiences as powerful and convincing as these women and have no doubt that homeopathy is an important personal tool for staying well. If you are new to homeopathy, you may have a 'try it and see' attitude. You will need careful guidance as to how to take the remedies, how often they are needed and the appropriate strengths. The addresses on page 255 may help you find a local homeopath. Training varies widely and anyone can adopt the title, so you will need to ask about the training and experience of any you choose.

The risks of homeopathic treatment

The Society of Homeopaths publishes a leaflet, *Homeopathy in Pregnancy and Childbirth*, in which they state than 'homeopathic remedies cannot cause side effects to either mother or baby' and can be used at the same time as treatment with orthodox drugs. Other homeopaths regularly remind the reader that their remedies are completely safe. This may be true of dilutions above 24X (or 12C) because these preparations contain no molecules from the original toxic substance used to make the remedy. However, below 12X (a measurement of concentration that reflects how many times the original substance is diluted), some of the original substance remains. Because the substances used are poisonous, many practitioners use only the higher dilutions in pregnancy. As homeopathic theory says that the more the preparation is diluted, the more powerful the effect, this seems not to get in the way of the therapy.

I have also known women who decided to use only external preparations during pregnancy. Calendula cream, tropical arnica preparations, and hypercal are all said to be helpful.

༄

Aromatherapy

Care should be taken if you use concentrated essential oils which are absorbed through the skin, either by massage or in the bath. Some oils should be avoided because they are thought to cause uterine bleeding, to be toxic or to carry the risk of inducing miscarriage or raising blood pressure.

Essential oils which should not be used in pregnancy:

Uterine bleeding	basil, camphor, clary sage, cypress, juniper, jasmine, hyssop, lavender, marjoram, myrrh, nutmeg, peppermint, rose, rosemary	hypertensive	sage, rosemary, hyssop, black pepper
Miscarriage	mugwort, pennyroyal, plecantrus, rue, savin, sage, tansy, thuja, wormwood	increased photo-sensitivity of the skin to sunlight	bergamot, tangerine, lemon and other citrus oils
Oestrogen-stimulating	aniseed, fennel		
Carcinogenic	basil, sassafras, terragon		
toxic	boldo, horseradish, mustard, wormseed		
moderately toxic	bitter almond, clove, hyssop, myrrh, parsleyseed, oregano, savory, thyme, whitegreen		

Source: Complimentaries in Pregnancy and Childbirth

129

The issue of using essential oils for expectant mothers needs more research before we can say definitely what is safe and which oils may affect the development of the baby.

⌘

In conclusion

You will probably follow what feels right for you when it comes to alternative remedies. By sharing with your doctor what you do and why you choose to do it, you may stimulate him or her to take a more curious and open-minded approach to all the options open to pregnant women. You may also alert him or her to anything that might be incompatible with your antenatal care, though there is little information about how alternative therapies and prescribed drugs might interact. Several books suggest a gap of two or three hours between taking herbs and any prescribed drugs. As far as I can tell, you would only put your baby at risk if you took herbs known to be dangerous or used these therapies instead of mainstream treatment, rather than in addition to it.

❧ 12 ❧

Alcohol in Pregnancy

Since a 'safe' limit for alcohol consumption during pregnancy has been set, your safest option is probably not to drink any alcohol in pregnancy. You have probably come across this advice many times before, yet you may not realize how recently it began to be the most common advice given to pregnant women. In 1980 when my friend Kathleen had her baby, her doctor suggested she drink a bit of sherry before bedtime to help her sleep. Ten years on, he is probably telling women to be teetotal from the moment they think about starting a baby until the baby is weaned. This chapter looks at why this has happened and what the consequences of the change are for women and babies. Has it changed what women do and how they feel? Have babies' chances of normal development and good health improved? And what about your own drinking – does your drinking or your partner's put your baby at risk? As you might expect, none of these questions have an easy answer.

Alcohol – the taboo of the 1990s

You would never guess that abstinence is a recent development from how fiercely some women take it up. A few months ago, I was at a party when the host offered wine to a guest. She gasped, 'I'm eight weeks pregnant!' as if just being close to alcohol might be dangerous. Her reaction clearly showed that

131

something quite powerful had shaped her view of alcohol. It reminded me of women I knew when I worked in West Africa. They, too, avoided certain things when they were pregnant – in one case, chicken and in another, certain local vegetables. When I asked them why, they said such foods would harm their baby. I did not then (and I do not now) see any rational explanation for such behaviour. By not eating chicken, a woman was using magic to protect her child. So was that woman at the party.

People use magic when they don't feel able to control what might happen and they care what the outcome will be very much. The bigger the gap between what you *hope* will happen and what you *fear* might happen, the more likely people are to turn to magic. Pregnancy and labour are like that – there is a huge gap between hopes and fears, and no way to be *sure* that the good ones happen and the bad ones don't. Anthropologists have found pregnancy and birth fertile ground for studying magic rituals and taboos.

Anthropologists tell us that it is not just those living in primitive tribes who use ritual and taboo during pregnancy and birth, we all do it. It is just as fruitful to study the birth rituals of Texan obstetricians as those of traditional birth attendants in Bali. Both have magic practices to control anxiety and tension. For example, doctors and midwives used to insist that men who wanted to be with their wives in labour wore special clothes and face masks. This was especially common when men were just starting to be allowed in and staff felt uneasy about their presence. One way to make the *staff* more comfortable was to ask men to wear this 'ritual' dress! Of course, quasi-rational explanations were offered about cleanliness and sterility but these had no basis in fact. Doctors came and went with their street shoes, fathers wore booties. And as staff have become more comfortable with the fathers, the ritual was dropped.

New rituals and taboos keep cropping up all the time. In the 1990s, *not* drinking is a pregnancy ritual. It marks a woman out as different long before it shows to the wider world, just as the booties did for fathers. Sometimes both partners abstain before conception and their decision announces their new status to friends and family. Other pregnancy rituals involve avoiding things – certain foods or sex perhaps – because to do otherwise would be seen as foolishness. Everyday things become taboo and doctor and woman alike shy away from them. Here's a leading American obstetrician in a book on preconceptual care:

> A recent study of coffee consumption in 12,000 women did not reveal any relationship between prematurity or malformation and coffee consumption – once the impact of cigarette smoking was considered ... I tell my patients attempting conception or already pregnant to cut coffee down to one cup per day, drink weak tea, cut out medication with caffeine and watch for excess cola consumption.

What's going on? The doctor admits he has no basis for making recommendations, then he proceeds to give arbitrary (one cup of coffee) or unspecific ('excess cola') orders to the reader. Is this because he feels that abstinence per se is good for her? Is this because the reader is anxious and wants to be given rules which help her feel safe? We do not know, but it has all the trappings of a taboo.

Alcohol is another very common taboo substance. People who favour the alcohol taboo (and that includes most practising obstetricians and, according to one survey, 89 per cent of educated, middle-class women) would say all this ethnographic chat was irrelevant. Chicken have not been shown to harm babies *in utero*. Neither, despite several studies (see page 119) has caffeine (unless consumed in excessive amounts). Alcohol clearly does when pregnant women drink excessively. But debate continues whether there is a safe limit and so at what level it should be set. It is better to err on the side of caution but, maybe it is only better when there is a danger in the first place. The real issue is whether the alcohol taboo keeps women from dangerous actions and spares babies; or whether it creates the perception of danger where none exists. In your particular case, you will not be able to judge this unless you look at your own drinking pattern. Does your drinking put your baby at risk?

ॐ

Alcohol and pregnancy – the continuing story

There is no doubt that a mother who drinks heavily (what constitutes 'heavy drinking' is explained below) puts her baby at much greater risk of abnormal development and retarded growth. Anti-alcohol campaigners have blamed alcohol for afflictions in the newborn for two centuries, although doctors have been slower to acknowledge the link between heavy drinking and abnormal babies. In her book *Women, Drinking, and Pregnancy*, Moira Plant quotes an American doctor who wrote in 1942, 'The belief that intoxication at the time of procreation may cause damage to the child ... has maintained itself up to the present time. On the basis of present knowledge, however, it may be dismissed.' (Plant notes that the doctor gives no hint of what this 'present knowledge' might be.) Similar reassuring statements recur through the 1960s. These 'experts' were *wrong*.

Advice to women began changing after two papers were published in medical journals in 1970 and 1973. In them, researchers describe the physical and mental characteristics of children born to alcoholic mothers. They claim that 30 per cent of these children showed a cluster of abnormalities which included failure to grow well before and after birth, abnormal brain development and characteristic changes in the shape of the baby's face and skull. These papers claimed that the features were so distinctive that a new syndrome – the Fetal Alcohol Syndrome or FAS – should be designated. Babies with FAS have at least one feature in each of the three following categories:

- *poor growth before and after birth* – small-for-date and failure to thrive (which may be related to poor maternal diet)
- *physical anomalies* – short, upturned nose, small eyes, receding chin and forehead, cleft palate, asymmetrical ears.
- *central nervous system problems* – learning difficulties, hearing and visual disabilities, and may also have congenital heart defects.

Those with the full syndrome seem likely to be mentally retarded, hyperactive, irritable, impulsive, unable to concentrate and to have social and behavioural problems later on. If one included children showing only one or two of these characteristics, 70 per cent of children born to alcoholic mothers were affected. Less acutely affected babies have been discussed as having Fetal Alcohol Effects (FAE), often with intellectual problems but without the facial symptoms.

This stimulated a flood of further investigations. Over a thousand papers have been published about the effects of alcohol on developing babies. Much of this research has gone into discovering whether or not alcohol-related damage goes up steadily as the amount a woman drinks increases. No such clear dose-response ratio has been found. One of the problems in assessing the evidence is separating the effects of alcohol from other factors such as diet, smoking, race and class, and we still do not know how to determine what level of drinking is harmful for each individual woman and her baby. The MIDIRS (see page 257) and NHS 1996 publication Alcohol and Pregnancy gives some helpful guidelines, defining drinking at three levels and relating these to units of alcohol and to possible risks:

- *Social drinking* is defined as less than ten units a week, and research suggests that for women who drink less than this number of units there is no evidence of fetal harm – provided that the drinking is spread over several days and not drunk all the time.
- *Frequent drinkers* are women who drink more than ten units a week but are not alcohol dependent. These women may be

at risk of giving birth to a baby with a number of individual abnormalities or FAE. These effects include heart, urogenital and brain abnormalities as well as behavioural disorders. But there is not much consistency or an identifiable problem in the features described for FAE, and these abnormalities remain controversial.

- *Alcohol dependent women* – those drinking more than three ounces of absolute alcohol or twelve units a day, are one in four to one in fifty depending on other factors (see p 137).

The evidence for an association between alcohol consumption and miscarriage is conflicting, although some researchers have suggested that heavy drinkers are more likely to have a miscarriage.

DEFINITION OF ONE UNIT OF ALCOHOL:

one pub measure of spirits
one pub glass of table wine
half pint of strong beer or cider
quarter pint of strong beer or lager

Remember that measures of alcohol you pour at home
may be larger than those in a pub or restaurant

In other words, if some women had one or two glasses of wine a day and some had none at all, they would all have the same chance of delivering a baby free of damage by alcohol. If they have more than ten units a week, the risk curve does start to rise slowly, but it does not increase sharply until a woman drinks more than three ounces of absolute alcohol a day (about 12 measures of spirits, 12 glasses of wine or 6 pints of beer or cider). At that point, it rises very steeply and this reflects the extreme dangers of alcoholic drinking.

Several other factors besides the daily amount have been shown to influence the amount of risk for the developing baby. These are:

- *when you drink* – Drinking heavily in the first third of pregnancy specially between the fifth and eleventh weeks, when the baby's organs are forming, carries a significantly higher chance of delivering a baby with abnormal face and skull development. A heavy drinker helps her baby by cutting down regardless of the stage of pregnancy she has reached. Giving up drinking in the second and last third of pregnancy has little effect on physical abnormalities but it does result in fewer underweight babies.
- *how often you drink* – Some studies show an increased risk where women drink seven or eight days out of ten.
- *your age* – The babies of older 'risk drinkers' fare worse than those of younger ones.
- *your race* – Black babies, for some unknown reason, carry seven times the risk of White babies, for the same amount of alcohol, so Black women need to be especially careful not to indulge in risk drinking.
- *how much you weigh* – the same quantity of alcohol will have a stronger effect on women who weigh less.
- *other risk factors in your lifestyle* – A poor diet, smoking, other drugs and having many children have been shown to increase the risks of damage from drinking.
- *binge drinking* – Binges in women who are already drinking heavily greatly increase the chances of a FAS baby. Binges in more abstemious women are the subject of the next section.

It may be hard to look honestly at the amount you drink. If you are a heavy drinker or carry any of the other risk factors listed above, you will help yourself have a healthier baby if you cut down or stop drinking. That is easy to say but may be very hard to do. Help, support and encouragement from those around you will help but only you can decide if the effort is worthwhile.

ↄ

The dangers of binge drinking

The chances are high that most of us will have a drink during or immediately before pregnancy, because alcohol is part of our lives. ('I love that moment when I get home from work, flop into a chair with a glass of red wine, and put on some music.') No one can say that a bit of alcohol in pregnancy is completely safe, but there is little evidence to support the position that alcohol (as opposed to *too much* alcohol) is dangerous. To think that every drink in some way diminishes the baby a tiny bit from what he or she might have otherwise been is a common misinterpretation of the facts. I remember the woman who said:

> I'm in business and I work hard and travel a lot. Last year, I had to close an important contract up North and I worried about it so much that when I got the deal of course we celebrated. In the evening, I accepted two gins – something I almost never do. The week after, I found I was six weeks pregnant. Those two drinks have ruined my pregnancy ... they have! I just can't stop worrying about what I did to the baby ...

Two gins is one thing; binge drinking is another matter. A 'binge' usually means drinking enough alcohol to make you feel drunk in a fairly short period of time. Experts vary in what they term 'a binge'. One said that three ounces of absolute alcohol would place a normally abstemious woman in a higher risk category, although, because women vary so much, less alcohol in some women may produce the same result. We do not really know the extent of risk if an occasional drinker drinks to the point of drunkenness on one occasion in early pregnancy.

Some researchers have suggested that if you drink enough quickly, enough to cause a surge of alcohol to flood your system, around the time of conception, in either the father or the mother, it could damage egg or sperm. If it happens between about the fourth and tenth week of your baby's life (that's the sixth to the twelfth week after your last period started), it could alter the way the baby develops. But again we do not really know.

Many women binge and many more worry about it. Ten per cent of women in Britain aged 18 to 24 report drinking three or more drinks every day. Many of us do not know when we conceive and we continue to drink like this. If you feel you might have placed your baby at risk because of binge drinking, you will naturally want to know how high the risk might be. But unfortunately, no one can tell you because people vary so much in their vulnerability to alcohol damage. Some of us seem to inherit a low threshold to alcohol damage; others possibly have the opposite tendency and can cope with a higher dosage without signs of damage. One journal reports the case of twins born to an alcoholic mother where one showed all the signs of alcohol damage and the other much less so.

Whatever your particular risk, though it is higher than it would be without that binge, it is still quite low. Alcohol damage, despite all the grim things described in this chapter, is rare in the general population. Sources vary but fetal alcohol syndrome (the full FAS with all the defects) is thought to occur about once or twice in a thousand births. All the women who have these babies will be drinking 'alcoholically' (they will be consuming way above the one ounce threshold already mentioned as designating risk). The literature does consider what are known as Fetal Alcohol Effects – a collection of physical conditions that appear to be more frequent in heavy drinkers. There is some evidence that a binge will increase a woman's chances of giving birth to a baby with one or more of these characteristics. Longitudinal studies show that these babies grow and behave normally.

Though the odds for social drinkers who sometimes exceed safe limits are not very high, especially in well-nourished generally healthy women, they seem to be higher in women who also smoke or have a poor diet. However, the worry that even the small increase in risk causes can be acute. And it can last well beyond the baby's birth. I remember a woman who, even as she held her normal six week old son, said, 'Do you think Simon's all right? He was conceived on a holiday in Spain and it was a pretty boozy few weeks'. She could see that his body was perfect but worried about his brain – could that have been damaged?

No one can say that there was no effect. After all, who can say what Simon's brain *would* have been like had his parents been teetotal? It makes no sense to measure this child against some mythical yardstick of 'perfection'. If his mother unconsciously changes the way she treats him because she assumes that he is subtly 'damaged', we know from other studies that this will influence how he grows. We simply know too little to judge the effects of binge drinking on normal babies like Simon.

꒰ꉂ

The origins of the blanket ban

So why, if there is little evidence to show that the occasional drink is not dangerous, do we see the ubiquitous advice to abstain from drinking in pregnancy? It's based on the fact that no one can extrapolate backwards from what is an accepted danger threshold, to one which is guaranteed to be safe. Given this uncertainty, banning it altogether makes doctors and mothers themselves feel better. As we saw in Chapter 4, doctors have good reasons for feeling uncomfortable unless they 'play it safe'. In 1981, that wariness reached new heights when the US Surgeon General recommended that women inspect foods and medicines to determine if they contain alcohol and, if so, avoid them. This has more to do with taboo and litigation than teratology.

Women who abstain from alcohol may go to equally great lengths. One of my friends refused Christmas pudding because of the brandy butter, and behaving like this is one way of taking control. Most women, in the heart of hearts, know they are helpless to ward off many dangers. One individual can do nothing about lead in petrol, Chernobyl, or the pesticide residues in the food we eat. As the head of the American Environmental Protection Agency remarked, 'We must now assume that life takes place in a minefield of hundreds of risks from thousands of substances.' He monitors the risks in a country where 25,000 chemicals are in regular use and between 700 and 3000 new ones are synthesized each year. Only a handful are ever tested as to their effect on a developing fetus. We do not know their effect and we cannot avoid them. 'You have to eat, you have to breathe … what can I do about it?' Not much. But you can say 'No' to a glass of wine and gain a sense of control and satisfaction. A teetotal women can feel she has made a small contribution towards her baby's good.

꒰

The cost of a blanket ban on alcohol

Some would argue that banning alcohol is no bad thing. After all, alcohol is implicated in domestic violence, football hooliganism, chronic disease, unwanted pregnancy … the list goes on. We would all be better off, both individually and as a society, if we drank less or not at all. As one director of an alcohol abuse programme pointed out, 'What is the great benefit of drinking at all? That's what people should be asking themselves, rather than this frantic search for a safe level.' So why not keep on suggesting the absolute ban on alcohol in pregnancy? Because there is too high a price to pay for the possible benefits to a few, in terms of worry and guilt in the many.

Like many other examples from obstetrics, a policy or treatment that is of real benefit to a small proportion of pregnant women does not benefit all pregnant women when it is applied to the group as a whole. Five per cent of women drink more than one ounce of absolute alcohol every day and are putting their babies at risk. There is little evidence that health warnings have changed their behaviour and it is not hard to see why. One or two women in every 100 in Britain (eight per 100 in the USA) are addicted – they are alcoholics who need specialized care urgently. They need more than 'Stop' to get them to cut down. They need sensitive, non-judgmental help.

Heavy drinkers are now harder to help than before so much attention was focused on alcohol and pregnancy. They probably lie about their drinking to themselves and others more than ever and they may even drink more to cope with their guilt. Stigmatizing women who drink heavily discourages them from seeking treatment early and some from coming forward at all. When they do come forward, painting the dangers with too broad a brush means that health workers do not focus their efforts on the 5 per cent who really need it.

Nor do health warnings help the 95 per cent of all pregnant women who were light or 'social' drinkers anyway, and who have not been shown to be at risk. They may even harm this group. Social drinkers can blame themselves if an abnormal child is born, whereas, in fact, the abnormality had nothing to do with their drinking. Even more tragically, family and friends can blame a mother on the same grounds.

Pregnancies can be marred by worry and an American doctor reports that one of his patients had an abortion following 'a bit of beer drinking'. All this blame, guilt and worry add up to a high price for warning the 95 per cent who are probably at little or no risk anyway. Two experts in the field of alcohol and pregnancy, Drs Rosette and Weiner, finish their book on alcohol and pregnancy with a plea for *realistic* counselling by doctors:

A woman should be given the opportunity to make informed decisions based on current medical evidence. When a mother assumes responsibility for deciding which risks she is willing to tolerate, she gains a sense of mastering her own life and a sense of personal freedom. This reduces stress, improves her chances of having a happy and healthy pregnancy, and lessens resentment that her baby caused her to abandon her normal life activities … For the most cautious, abstention removes all danger from alcohol; there seems to be no harm from not drinking. However, the recommendation that all women should refrain from drinking in pregnancy is not based on scientific evidence since no risks have been observed from consumption of small amounts (never exceeding 1 oz of absolute alcohol or 1–2 drinks per day). Issuing health recommendations that cannot be demonstrated as fact helps legitimize unproven, superstitious health fads …

And a professor of obstetrics has recently said 'women with a modest intake such as those who are occasional social drinkers should be reassured that one or two drinks a day carries a negligible risk … The pregnant woman has enough to worry about without being burdened with worry and possible guilt about negligible risks'.

Both parents can look at how much they drink and if necessary cut right down. Unless either drinks very heavily or binges in the first third of pregnancy, they should not assign any responsibility for damage to their own baby to their drinking.

∾ 13 ∾

Smoking in Pregnancy

It ought to be easy to write a chapter on smoking in pregnancy – you just tell women that smoking harms the baby and suggest they stop. It is not that women are not aware of the dangers. In one survey carried out by the Health Education Authority in 1993 almost 90 per cent of women asked considered smoking to be dangerous to the unborn child, and some do give up during pregnancy. But it isn't that easy or 28 per cent of pregnant women in Britain would not still be smoking cigarettes. So instead, this chapter sets out to explore what we know about the effects of smoking on pregnancy and on the baby, and how (if you smoke) you can use this information to gather up your courage and stop.

∾

The case against smoking in pregnancy

Advice to pregnant women usually lumps smoking and drinking together and suggests strongly that you avoid both. But the case against tobacco is much stronger. We can be certain that smoking *causes* harm to the mother, the placenta and the baby and it seems that it exacerbates the risks of caffeine and alcohol.

- We know that smoking – any amount of smoking – is detrimental to the baby's health.
- We know how the chemicals and gases in cigarettes cause harmful changes in the mother, the placenta and the baby.
- In general, the effects of cigarettes are dose-related (the more you smoke, the more likely it is you will be harmed and the more serious the harm).
- We can predict effects on the baby if we know how much the mother smokes. These predictions are not always correct but the chances that a baby will be smaller than he should be, are easier to predict if you know how much a woman smokes than if you know other facts about her, such as income, race, alcohol intake or nutritional state.

The evidence about smoking is vast. In the last 35 years, thousands of papers, hundreds of books and scores of international symposia have come to the same conclusion: that smoking is harmful in pregnancy and that the babies of smokers fare worse than those born to non-smokers. However, there is little evidence that this research has been translated into clinical practice. In one study, only 19 per cent of GPs even mentioned smoking to their pregnant patients. And in the last 20 years, the percentage of pregnant women who smoke has not fallen.

This is despite the fact that we know that people who smoke will be healthier if they stop. That is true if you are pregnant and it is equally true if you are not pregnant. Anyone who lives with someone who smokes would be healthier if the other person stops, because of the dangers of passive smoking. But just knowing this is not enough. Health arguments alone do no change people's actions (though convincing women there is a risk is an important first step). Pregnant smokers, like all smokers, may be addicted and the ones who continue to smoke are highly likely to be so. They need help, support and encouragement to stop and, sadly, this has been singularly lacking in the last 25 years of health education directed at pregnant women. Instead they get scare tactics, blame and guilt – none of which has worked. This chapter finishes by examining what might help you smoke less or stop altogether – for your own sake and your baby's.

⤳

Who smokes in pregnancy?

Worldwide, one child in five is born to a smoking woman. This number is rising because developing countries show increases in their smoking rates which are greater than the rate of population growth. In developed countries, more women under twenty take up smoking than men, and in all age groups, women are slower to give up the habit than men. All this means that more and more babies will be conceived by men and women who smoke, many of whom will continue to do so.

Only a third of smokers stop once they know they are pregnant. Those who do either see pregnancy as a spur for kicking a habit they wanted to be of anyway or they suddenly find cigarettes unpalatable and simply stop. About 40 per cent of British women begin pregnancy as smokers; 10 per cent stop early in the pregnancy and 30 per cent continue to smoke.

Even if the mother does not smoke, the baby may be exposed to cigarette smoke through passive smoking. About 60 per cent of households have at least one smoker and many women work in a smoky atmosphere. The evidence about passive smoking is less clear-cut than that for primary smokers but anyone who lives or works in a smoky atmosphere is said to inhale the equivalent of 14 cigarettes a day. If this applies to you, you can mentally substitute the word 'passive' before every reference to smokers in the rest of the chapter. Unfortunately, much less effort has gone into helping passive smokers become smoke-free because convincing someone else to stop or pressing your employer to safeguard your environment are both difficult although attitudes have started to change in the past few years and smoking at work and in public places is becoming less acceptable. At work, your union representative may be the best place to start.

჻

Smoking and conception

If you are planning a pregnancy, you are more likely to conceive a baby if you and your partner stop smoking. One study showed that non-smoking women aged 20 to 29 took, on average, six months to conceive; those smoking twenty cigarettes a day took 9.6 months; and those smoking 40 a day took 11.2 months. Another report, in the medical journal the *Lancet* in 1992 suggested that smokers were three and a half times more likely than non-smokers to have taken more than a year to conceive.

No one is sure exactly why this delay occurs. One possibility is that smoking delays the surge of hormones needed to trigger the release of the egg. Or it may be that the partners of these women were smokers and the delay was caused by a decrease in the male hormone, testosterone, a reduction in sperm concentration, or an increase in the percentage of abnormal sperm caused by smoking. One author speculates that the egg is less likely to implant because the low oxygen levels and nicotine in the bloodstream change the environment in the uterus. It could be that all these as well as other unknown factors are involved. Whatever the cause of delayed conception, most pre-pregnancy clinics recommend that both partners stop smoking some months before they try to conceive, and they certainly suggest that any couple having trouble conceiving do so. Stopping smoking appears to return fertility to that of 'never smokers'.

If you conceived a baby while you were still smoking and have since stopped, you may worry that this harmed the baby. The good news is that tobacco smoke does not appear to be a strong teratogen – that is, babies born to smokers do not seem to have rates of congenital abnormality which are any higher than that of babies born to non-smokers. However, a recent survey in Hungary found that there was an association between smoking in pregnancy and congenital limb defects, and another study in the USA found a higher risk of congenital urinary tract anomalies.

Smoking is believed to cause harm not by interfering with the normal pattern of cell development but by inhibiting normal cell *growth* and changing how the placenta grows and develops. By stopping early in pregnancy, you avoid this first complication, and by stopping soon after conception, you minimize any changes in the placenta, although you do not eliminate them.

However, there is some evidence that smoking, while not a strong teratogen, can cause subtle changes to the egg and sperm which, fused together, create a baby. It may also alter how the cells develop. Most of our knowledge about smoking around conception comes from animal studies and these show that smoking does damage sperm and increase the risk of damage to the egg. Any resulting embryo will be abnormal and thus, more likely to miscarry. If this is true in humans too, this may be one reason why smokers have double the risk of miscarriage when compared to non-smokers.

Smoking in pregnancy may also have longer term effects on the baby. A study in Sweden found that childhood cancers were 50 per cent more common in children whose mothers smoked throughout pregnancy and childhood. And an American study reported in 1991 concluded that the risk for all cancers was 30 per cent higher for the children of mothers who had smoked in pregnancy. The research does not show that prenatal smoking *causes* cancers but it does show that children of smokers are more prone to developing them. Smoking during pregnancy has also been associated with a higher risk of serious respiratory illness, such as bronchitis, asthma and pneumonia, and some researchers have suggested that this is because exposure to cigarette smoke in the womb affects the lungs of the baby. Smoking also seems to increase the risk of 'glue ear', one of the commonest causes of deafness in young children.

ᴄᴏ

Smoking and pregnancy

At all stages of pregnancy, smokers have a higher risk of complications than non-smokers. These are probably caused, at least in part, by changes in the placenta. Smokers tend to have larger placentas, probably as a compensation for lower oxygen levels in the mother's blood, but these bulky placentas work less efficiently than those of non-smokers and they are further compromised by several of the thousands of chemicals and gases found in tobacco smoke. Many of these can cross the placenta, and two which are thought to be very significant are: *carbon monoxide*, a gas that interferes with oxygen-carrying capacity of the blood; and *nicotine*, a chemical that constricts the arteries bringing blood to the placenta.

Smokers experience:

- a greater risk of ectopic pregnancy
- more episodes of bleeding in pregnancy
- a greater risk of miscarriage
- a greater risk that the placenta will separate from the wall of the uterus. On average, nine women in 10,000 who are non-smokers suffer sudden and complete separation of the placenta from the wall of the uterus, placing the mother's life at risk from haemorrhage and nearly always costing the baby's life. This happens to 25 women in 10,000, who smoke twenty cigarettes a day.
- more risk that the membranes will rupture prematurely
- and more risk that the baby will be born too early

ᴄᴏ

Smoking and prematurity

The relationship between cigarette smoking and prematurity is a complicated one. We do not know exactly how smoking causes the membranes to rupture or how smoking causes babies to be born early, but the two events – smoking and prematurity – happen together much more often than you would expect by chance. One retrospective study (one that starts with premature babies and then looks backwards at the characteristics of those babies' mothers) looked at very premature babies, born between 20 and 32 weeks. The study found such babies were 60 per cent more common among smoking mothers than non-smokers. For every 100 premature babies born to non-smokers, 160 were born to smokers.

The trouble with interpreting data like this is that women who smoke may be more likely to do other things that might cause a baby to be born prematurely. For example, a recent study in Inner London found that smoking *per se* was not associated with prematurity, but that adverse social circumstances were. It is hard to untangle how important a factor smoking is compared to others when deciding what caused a particular baby to be premature. But we do know that women who smoke have more premature babies than women who do not smoke. And women who smoke more than 20 cigarettes a day are more likely to have premature babies than women who smoke less than 20 cigarettes a day. One doctor, drawing conclusions from these findings, claimed that for every 100 babies born before 37 weeks, four came early simply because their mother smoked. For those born before 33 weeks, nine could be attributed directly to smoking.

∾

Smoking and its effect on the baby

Smoking stunts a baby's growth before birth: researchers have found a direct relationship between the number of cigarettes smoked and the amount of weight the baby should have gained but did not (this is assessed by measuring the ratio between the baby's length and weight) and it is found regardless of what kind of cigarette the mother smoked, or how deeply she inhaled. The only thing that mattered was how many cigarettes she smoked a day.

One study found the mothers who smoked between one and six cigarettes a day gave birth to babies who weighed, on average, 88 grams less than babies born to mothers who differed only in that they did not smoke. Women smoking fourteen or more per day had babies weighing 248 grams less than women who did not smoke. Dozens of other studies produced similar results and it is estimated that smoking decreases average birth weight by 200 grams and doubles the risk of low birth weight.

Fathers who smoked also had babies who were smaller than they should have been. A Danish study found that there was almost as much effect on the birth weight from male smoking as from female. On average, the babies weighed 6.1 grams less from every cigarette he smoked in a day, totalling around 250 grams. This is very close to the total found in studies for women, and it could either be the result of passive smoking by the mother or changes in sperm around the time of conception.

What is a pregnant woman to make of the information that if she smokes, her baby will be smaller than it should be? Does it make any difference? The next section tries to answer these questions.

Understanding the statistics

When given facts about how smoking retards a baby's growth, pregnant women react in two very different ways. Many disregard the news. If you tell a mother her baby will be smaller than it should be, you are almost guaranteed to hear stories about her sister who smoked and had an eight pound baby; or about the birth weights of her other children. The smoker is saying, 'See! Your statistics don't apply to me.'

Some women welcome the news that smoking interferes with a baby's growth – a small baby is an easy birth. This is a fantasy because births involving tiny babies are no easier than those of good-sized ones. A midwife who regularly meets this attitude said to me in exasperation, 'I want to ask them how they would feel about a mother who underfed her toddler and denied him milk, so she wouldn't have to spend so much on new clothes because he outgrew the old ones. I can't see how it's all that different from what they do by smoking, but I keep quiet so as not to offend them.'

Other mothers, on hearing the case against smoking, are more concerned and ask questions like 'Does it matter that my baby will weigh a bit less? Eighty grams isn't all that much ...' 'Will it make any difference if I stop now? I'm sixteen weeks' and 'I know quitting will be agony for me. How can I be sure it will make things that much better for the baby?' These are complicated questions and they will take some unravelling before you might arrive at an answer.

Does it matter that cigarettes cause a decrease in the birth weight of affected babies? Yes, it matters, because all our babies deserve the best start they can have and these babies are not just small, they are stunted. We do not know exactly how these babies' growth was inhibited, but it is probably due to the effects of a cocktail of gases and chemicals, most of which are known to be poisons. It's a rotten atmosphere in which to start one's life.

But the growth retardation matters most of all because it is one more handicap for your baby in the journey towards good health that begins before conception and lasts through life. To see what this means, it may help to imagine that a baby enters a sort of race at conception which eventually has a finishing line marked 'maximum good health'. If the baby's mother is well-fed, well-housed, well-educated and well-supported by those around her, her baby can begin at the starting line because he or she carries few additional risks to his or her health. That does not mean a healthy mother will be sure of a healthy baby, it means that her baby faces no extra risks.

If, however, a healthy mother smokes, her baby is at more risk than if she does not. In the race, this baby starts back from the starting line and has to run harder to catch up. Most babies can cope with this with little trouble and we all know cases of mothers who smoked and gave birth to healthy (albeit some-what too small) babies. However, the more risks the mother's lifestyle contains, the farther back her baby begins. For some babies, it will be a race for life itself. A baby born to a mother who is anaemic, poor, undernourished, anxious and who has already lost one baby, must start 'running' well back from the starting line. Some of these babies manage to get there despite the hurdles; many don't.

This image of a race is born out by the statistics. Small babies are more likely to die and more likely to be ill. One study analysed the increased risk of a baby dying between the twenty-eighth week of pregnancy and the first week of life (called the Perinatal Mortality Rate) for babies whose mothers carried various combinations of risks – 52 in all. What was soon clear is that for some, the increased risks of smoking were quite small. For others, smoking nearly doubled the chances that a baby would die.

If you are a mother who has no other risk factors, the increased risk to your baby of smoking twenty cigarettes a day is about 10 per cent. That means that if a thousand ordinary women who did not smoke had babies, we would expect around ten babies to die between the twenty-eighth week of pregnancy and the first week of life. But if they all smoked a pack a day, we would expect eleven to die.

The study also looked at women who were having their fourth child, were living on a very low income, had already had one premature baby and were anaemic. If these women also smoked more than a pack a day, they had a 70 per cent increased risk of the baby dying. So, if 1000 such women gave birth, we would expect higher perinatal mortality among their babies anyway – say 15 babies. If, using the same ratio, these high-risk women also smoked, as many as 26 could die, and many more would be poorly, because those 26 simply could not cope with the extra handicaps arising from their mother's lifestyles.

A more recent study in Sweden of 280,000 births also showed that maternal smoking significantly increased the risk of perinatal death.

Smoking has also been associated with sudden infant death syndrome (cot death), although the evidence is not unequivocal and different studies have shown conflicting results. By smoking, you have not condemned your baby to ill-health or death, but you have increased the chances. Only you can decide whether or not to add this extra risk to your baby's life and health.

~

Thinking about stopping?

I suspect anyone reading the last few pages would at least *think* about giving up cigarettes. Even supposing the risk to your baby is small compared to the risks run by other women, and even though smoking is not the only thing that compromises a baby's health, *not* smoking is a positive step towards a healthy life that you can give your baby. It is one risk factor you can do something about.

Regardless of the risks your baby faces, he or she will benefit if you stop, and the earlier in pregnancy you do, the greater the benefit. Here's some evidence to show this is so.

- There is no difference in the number of low birth weight babies born to women who never smoked, women who used to smoke and women who stop smoking before pregnancy or during the first twelve weeks of pregnancy. The evidence about the impact of *cutting down* on smoking and birth weight is less clear.
- Women who stop after 16 weeks and anytime before 30 weeks have babies that are smaller than non-smokers but larger than those born to women who keep on smoking throughout their pregnancy.
- Even after 24 weeks, babies can recover from weight loss caused by smoking. The evidence for this comes from the fact that the best way to predict the decrease in birth weight is to measure the amount smoked in the last third of pregnancy.

- Your baby will even benefit if you stop two days before a Caesarian section, because babies who have even two days free from cigarette smoke have higher oxygen levels at birth than those who have no break. One study showed that even if smoking is stopped for only 48 hours there is an 8 per cent rise in available oxygen for the baby.
- It would help your baby if you stopped an hour before birth because then he or she would grow up in a smoke-free home and there is evidence that passive smoking harms children.

It is never too late to stop but that is not the only way you can help your baby. While you decide about stopping, you could smoke less. Almost all the studies show that the damage caused by cigarettes is dose-related. That is, the more you smoke, the worse it is for your baby, so the less you smoke, the better. You could smoke half the number, half the cigarette, none before noon ... whatever might work for you. The longer the gap between cigarettes, the more time your baby has to recover from the effects.

You could consider using patches or chewing gum to help you give up, although the use of replacement therapies is 'contraindicated' in pregnancy, because the nicotine will still affect the baby. I could only find one study and this suggests that, if it helps you to give up, the benefits of nicotine replacement therapy outweigh the risks of continued smoking.

What about changing your diet? Many smokers clearly hope this will help. I read a library book about nutrition in pregnancy. One sentence was underlined: 'Only when the mother uses cigarettes as a substitute for good food does she run the risk of having a sickly baby.' The evidence to back up this sweeping statement does not exist though some guilty smoker clearly latched on to it. Good food does not remove all risk, though, of course, a poor diet will further increase the risk for mother and baby. Compensatory eating will make no difference to how the placenta grows nor will it alter chemical changes caused by the poisons in tobacco.

One step that will help is to acknowledge any guilt feelings you may have (most smokers do feel guilty), and do something about them. It might help keep your feelings in proportion by remembering that the risks to the baby vary according to the lifestyle of the mother, so remind yourself of the helpful things you do do for your baby, as well as the harmful ones. It could help to talk about your feelings with a sympathetic, non-judgmental listener. Or, best of all, you could try to stop smoking again.

If you go on feeling guilty and anxious, you may be even more likely to feel the need to smoke to calm you down. It could mean your body makes chemicals that will speed the baby's heart and this will narrow his or her arteries in much the same way as some of the chemicals in cigarettes do. Unfortunately, much of the educational material aimed at pregnant women over the past few decades is designed to induce guilt.

༈

The campaign against smoking in pregnancy

Until the early 1970s, anti-smoking campaigns were almost entirely targeted at men because, as they smoked more and had done so for longer, most of the health problems caused by smoking were showing up in men. Then someone noticed that women, too, were smoking in greater numbers and soon they, too, were suffering the ill effects of tobacco. So the health educators thought, 'Why not direct a campaign at women?'

The first female anti-smoking campaign focused on pregnant women: they were such an obvious target. Here was a distinct group which was known to face many changes and presumed to be motivated to change because of nurturing feelings towards the baby. If they could be convinced to stop, then that would help two people at once, and the evidence was strong that once stopped, most women continued to abstain up to a year after the birth.

The first campaigns aimed at women were based on two feelings: guilt and fear. One memorable film showed a worried mother standing beside an incubator in which a very tiny baby lay wired to machines. A slow male voice described how cigarette smoking kills babies. Posters implied that smoking mothers cared less about their babies than non-smokers. Not only were both claims unfair, they were also untrue. Even heavy smokers have live babies most of the time. An Australian study showed no difference in feelings of attachment among smokers who tried and failed to stop, as compared to those who did. Both groups felt as warmly towards their babies. What governed their behaviour was not mother-love, or lack of it, but addiction to nicotine.

These early campaigns and most that followed had no impact and the explanations why this was so are not hard to find. A campaign won't work if it:

- *over-sells the dangers of smoking* – Such an approach doesn't fit the personal experience of pregnant smokers and women simply don't believe it or deny it.
- *makes sweeping statements about all babies* – Because the risks are greater for women with multiple risk factors, and because these women are more likely to smoke, targeting the message will be more effective in reducing the number of damaged babies.
- *ignores the fact that cigarettes are addictive* – Realistic campaigns separate the facts about damage from the help and support an addicted person needs to stop. One does not follow automatically from the other.
- *does not acknowledge the special problems of stopping in pregnancy* – Some women find it easy to stop when pregnant so they need little help. The ones who continue find the anxieties and challenges of pregnancy make stopping even more difficult then than at other times and anxiety may even make them smoke more.

Women cannot be frightened or bullied or shamed into deciding to stop. To work, a campaign must go beyond the rational facts to acknowledge the feelings, fears and needs of pregnant smokers. It is easier to do difficult things if we feel good about ourselves and harder if we feel ashamed or undermined by our actions. This holds true for stopping smoking, too. We know from the experience of groups like ASH (see address on page 255) that women find giving up harder than men, but that the ones who manage it are usually those who plan ahead, get good support from those around them and who feel good about themselves, rather than guilty about their smoking. They give up for themselves and see the benefits to the baby as a bonus.

ༀ

A personal note

I was feeling very bogged down by the history of anti-smoking campaigns for pregnant women until I met Renate. Here's what she told me:

> I smoked all the time I was pregnant with Natalie, my first one, and felt terrible about it. I knew I should stop but life was too awful anyway without that, too. I was on my own, no proper house – all that. Then I met Micky and life got better bit by bit. Now I'm pregnant again and I'm determined to stop. My health visitor runs a special session to help pregnant women who smoke and I went along expecting a lecture. Well, we got some of that, but she asked us to write down all the good things we do for our children. It was like all of a sudden someone was saying, 'You *are* a good mother' which makes a change, doesn't it? I mean, Natalie's a smashing kid and I love her, and so many kids don't have that, and then I think about the new baby and try and remember that I am a good mother for that one, too. That was three weeks ago but I have picked a day for stopping – next Monday. This time, Micky wants me to, too ...

And she did ...

༚ 14 ༚

Street Drugs and Pregnancy

Reliable estimates about drug users are difficult to obtain, but many pregnant women do use illegal drugs occasionally or regularly, as part of their everyday lives.

Reports indicate that a growing number of babies are born to mothers using a variety of drugs. Information about what some street drugs do to women and babies can make grim reading. We need to know the real risks to mothers and babies so that these inform laws about drugs and influence professionals like social workers, health visitors and judges whose job it is to decide the future of babies born to drug-addicted mothers.

Some people argue that describing risks to occasional users is pointless because there are no benefits to balance them. However users need solid facts to help them to decide what to do, and motivation and support if they make up their minds to abstain. Non-users need good information, too, to make judgements about drugs based on reason rather than prejudice.

༚

Studying the problems

All studies of illicit drug use in pregnancy are fraught with difficulties and there is relatively little research, with the exception of US studies of cocaine use. In order to assess the risk of drug A, you need to know who is using it; how much she consumes; how often she does so; what difficulties crop up during her pregnancy; and how her baby differs from one born to a woman who is like her in many respects, but avoids drug A. Now that sounds straightforward enough but turns out to be tricky in practice, even if what you are studying is legal as we saw in Chapter 4. The problem multiplies when the substance is illegal because:

- Women who use illicit drugs may try to conceal this because they fear disapproval, feel guilty or worry that the baby will be taken away.
- Women and babies most at risk from damage due to illegal drugs are the hardest to find because they avoid antenatal care. They are also the easiest to lose in follow-up studies.
- Drug use is often associated with other risky habits and unhealthy lifestyles, any or all of which could have caused whatever abnormalities are detected and it is difficult to distinguish the effects of use of these drugs from other lifestyle factors such as smoking, alcohol or poor diet.
- Street drugs are adulterated with unknown substances and also used in various combinations where any or all of the substances could cause harm and it is hard to tell which might be responsible for a problem with the baby.

Dealing with the results

An interested observer, approaching the vast number of papers about illegal drugs, would find three things difficult:

1 *Searching out specific answers for specific questions.* You cannot find an answer to the kind of questions pregnant women ask like, 'Did the LSD we took just before I got pregnant have anything to do with our baby's heart murmur?' or 'Is it OK to smoke marijuana after the first twelve weeks?'

  Unless a drug is fairly popular in the group of women being studied, you will need to sample thousands to produce even a few who admit to being users. Many conclusions are based on a few cases; some on studies of a few dozen. With such small numbers, you can be sure that you have not over-looked a connection between cause and effect or that some-thing has not simply happened by chance. It takes many examples before researchers can conclude that the result is probably linked with the drug itself and not some other factor. Even with a few hundred users in a study, it will be difficult to tell the effect of taking the drug occasionally or regularly, taking it early or late in pregnancy, or taking it in large or small amounts.

2 *Deciding if the results apply to you.* For example, most studies of cocaine are done on addicts but far more women use the drug now and again and have a lifestyle vastly different from that of an addict. How do the conclusions based on addicted women apply to occasional users? Many studies are done with a clearly defined group of women rather than a cross section of the population. So how can you know if the results apply to you?

3 *Keeping a sense of proportion.* I spent two grim weeks reading dozens of papers about addiction in pregnancy. Then I met, as I regularly do, a group of pregnant women. I had to keep reminding myself that, even though anyone *could* be using illegal drugs regularly without my knowledge, I probably didn't have to regard them as potential addicts. Most women are their babies fiercest protectors rather than abusers.

That is not to say that there is not a problem – there is. In America, cocaine and 'crack' have reached epidemic propor-tions. Hospitals that cater for poor women living in large American cities now routinely test the urine of women in labour and some find that one woman in four is a cocaine user. Urban neonatal nurseries around the developed world are faced with caring for the babies of addicted mothers. We read newspaper articles about 'crack babies' and those who are HIV positive because their mothers have become infected through sharing needles or syringes.

The problem itself is growing but the papers studying the problem are also growing. In the 1990s, it is urban hospitals that find themselves in the front line. Doctors who work there need to write papers as part of their careers and they turn to the problems around them, filling the journals with articles about hard drug use. The advantage of this is that we are learning more about the effects of illegal drugs on babies. The disadvantage is that many health professionals will slip into the same state of misapprehension as I did. The challenge is to acknowledge the gravity of the problem, yet still keep a sense of proportion. It is noteworthy that a recent appraisal of research into the effects of cocaine showed that research reporting adverse effects was more likely to be published than that reporting an absence of such effects. While not denying the existence of adverse effects, there is a danger that over-emphasis may persuade some women to consider a termination when they perhaps need not.

Conclusions change rapidly and clear and reliable information is difficult to establish. However the following summary sets out some of what we know in general, and also in relation to specific drugs. Organizations such as SCODA and ISDD can provide more detailed information (see page 254).

For pregnant drug users in general, irrespective of the drugs used, there is an increased risk of:

- low birth weight baby
- perinatal mortality (death in the first week of life)
- congenital abnormalities, which for drug users are in the 'high normal' range (2.7–3.2 per cent of all pregnant drug users who give birth). The main risk period is probably the first three months of pregnancy
- sudden infant death syndrome.

ॐ

Amphetamines

Women who take amphetamines may increase the risk that their baby will develop abnormally or grow poorly although the dose and frequency that causes damage is unclear. Studies show that cleft hip or palate, heart deformities, and an abnormally small head are all more common and some researchers have suggested that maternal amphetamine abuse during pregnancy can also have long-term effects on children's mental and intellectual development. Babies are likely to be born too early and weigh less than babies born to non-users possibly because amphetamines act as an appetite suppressant. Ecstasy (MDMA) is an amphetamine derivative and although there are as yet no published case reports which implicate it in fetal damage, ecstasy and other forms of amphetamine should be avoided in pregnancy. Stopping taking amphetamines will not cause withdrawal and should stop as soon as you think you might be pregnant.

ॐ

Barbiturates

Massive doses of phenobarbitone in pregnancy have been associated with distortions of facial features and finger malformations.

ॐ

Cannabis

Smoking cannabis during pregnancy, either as 'grass' or in its more concentrated resin form, has not been linked with higher rates of abnormality in babies. One of the most extensive studies into the effects of cannabis on the fetus was of 700 women in Canada not from deprived backgrounds. One adverse effect was found. Heavy cannabis users gave birth, on average, a week earlier than women in the matched control group. Other smaller studies have shown a range of adverse outcomes, in particular low birth weight and prematurity, in babies of heavy cannabis smokers, but these studies have tended to involve women whose lifestyle and diet could also be factors.

Babies born to cannabis smokers behave differently than those born to unexposed women. Babies of heaviest users in the Canadian study startled more easily and took longer to become used to a light shone by the researcher. Several studies show that animals and humans exposed to large amounts of cannabis before birth were slower to reach developmental milestones but they offer no explanation as to why this might be.

One anomalous study caused quite a stir in scientific circles where researchers presume drug effects are going to be negative. This one showed that exposed infants did better than their counterparts. They scored higher on motor development, proved better at following an object with their eyes, and were judged more alert when tested at 12 weeks. Later, researchers decided these findings were flukes, based on too small a number to be regarded.

I regularly meet women who say they used cannabis and had a healthy baby ('I was living in Liberia and didn't know I was pregnant until I was five months. I smoked every day but Neil is fine'). However, the fact that cannabis changes the newborn's behaviour means that it does affect the baby, and animal studies with high levels of the drug do show problems. Prudence dictates caution and smokers are reminded that tobacco, so often linked with cannabis, is known to be detrimental to babies.

ح

Cocaine

Dr Barry Brazelton is a widely known American paediatrician who works in Boston. In a television interview, he summed up the evidence about cocaine in one sentence, 'Cocaine is real bad for babies.' It is also 'real bad' for mothers. Women who use cocaine regularly are more likely to miscarry and more likely to go into labour prematurely. Some studies find that cocaine users have higher rates of *abruptio placenta*, a condition where the placenta separates suddenly from the wall of the uterus, threatening the mother's life through bleeding and almost always causing the baby to die.

All these complications are probably caused by a sudden rise in blood pressure as cocaine clamps down the user's (and her baby's) blood vessels. Urban casualty departments regularly treat users for vascular collapse related to cocaine use. In less extreme cases, tight blood vessels deprive the placenta of blood so that sections of it die.

Cocaine passes quickly to the baby where it can act as a direct teratogen in the first twelve weeks of pregnancy. Heart, genital and urinary defects are more common in babies of regular users. Throughout pregnancy, cocaine interferes with normal growth by depriving the baby of food and oxygen. Babies are born lighter than they should be, they have smaller heads, or they are more likely to be stillborn. Because the baby's cells are quickly dividing and growing, they are very susceptible to being starved of oxygen and some cells will die when the mother takes the cocaine. Doctors in American urban hospitals are used to delivering babies with gangrenous fingers and toes. Dr Brazelton describes brain 'holes' in babies born to addicted mothers, caused by lack of oxygen.

Nor are these babies' troubles over once they are born. One recent finding is that some cocaine babies initially have visual problems. A study of 39 'crack babies' found that seventeen had abnormal brain tracings in the first week of life, nine were still abnormal in the second week and one baby had not recovered when he or she was retested at 12 months. 34 of the 39 babies in the study were described as 'very irritable'. It is a word that crops up in most studies of such babies. Cocaine seems to leave these babies' brains somehow disorganized, so the world seems a terrifying and frightening place. To help them you need immense patience and sensitivity and we are beginning to develop regimes that seem to work. Initially they may cry a lot and any stimulation makes them stiffen and scream. But, in time, these babies can be gently held and they can be helped to slowly make sense of the world.

Cocaine addiction is devastating for babies, but the number of women using cocaine now and again far outnumber those using it regularly. What are the risks for their babies? Some researchers have found that even 'light' users have a higher risk of miscarriage and premature delivery, whereas another study of social cocaine users who stopped when they realized they were pregnant concluded that the rate of adverse outcome was no worse than the general population. However it is probably safe to assume that even one dose of cocaine in early pregnancy may be teratogenic. At any time in pregnancy, the drug will subject a baby to a sudden loss of oxygen which could lead to damage or death of growing cells. It could also cause the placenta to separate abruptly from the uterus. Used around the time of labour, cocaine increases the chance that labour will be dangerously short, it makes abnormal heartbeats in the baby more common, and it increases the number of babies at risk of inhaling meconium, a substance normally kept in the baby's bowel until birth but passed when the baby is short of oxygen. All in all, cocaine is bad news for babies.

🔊

Heroin and methadone

The use of heroin and other opiates in pregnancy is associated with low birth weight and there is evidence of a link with fetal growth retardation. There have been no reports of congenital abnormalities as a result of heroin use in pregnancy.

The lifestyle of some heroin users may mean that their babies are subject to risks posed by poor diet and ill-health. Yet many receive no antenatal attention. Diseases including HIV/AIDS, hepatitis, and septicaemia are associated with injecting drug use and/or sharing equipment, posing a serious risk to the baby. Many babies born to heroin addicts show symptoms of drug withdrawal and need drug treatment to get over this time. These babies may be irritable, restless, have vomiting, diarrhoea, convulsions and feeding difficulties. With good help and support, these children can improve. The only good thing to say about babies born to heroin addicts is that they do better than those born to women taking methadone, a drug prescribed by doctors to stabilize addicts and gradually wean them from drugs.

Withdrawal from heroin and other opiates in pregnancy should be done slowly under medical supervision. Abrupt withdrawal is associated with premature labour and fetal distress and death. A clinician in Glasgow has however helped over 50 women to withdraw from heroin without substituting another drug and without any harm to the baby.

Methadone is legally available for registered addicts in Britain and the hope is that dispensing methadone frees users from the pressures and dangers of buying drugs illegally. It also brings addicts into contact with other services so that methadone mothers are much more likely to have some ante-natal care. They are less likely to be anaemic and more likely to keep in contact with professionals after birth.

Unfortunately, because methadone is taken regularly, by mouth, it accumulates much more readily in the baby than heroin. Children born to methadone users fare worse in any tests designed to measure physical and mental abilities at the time of birth. In time, these abnormal findings seem to fade, and by the age of two, they seem to function as well as contemporaries from similar backgrounds who were not exposed to methadone before birth. Recent studies conclude that no long-term developmental problems can be directly attributed to methadone alone.

༄

LSD

In the early studies of LSD, users were found to have broken and damaged chromosomes. Researchers speculated that this could happen to the egg and sperm destined to form a baby and lead to higher miscarriage rates and more abnormal babies. Subsequent studies do not substantiate this fear. The breaks proved to be only temporary and rates of abnormality were not found to be higher than the population as a whole. Miscarriage rates were higher than expected only in women who use illicit LSD and not in those given the drug for psychiatric reasons which was done in the 1960s and 1970s.

Pregnant women are still advised to be cautious. This drug has a powerful effect on the adult brain and it is still not clear what changes it makes in the baby. A further risk comes from unknown contaminants in illicit drugs. One woman who used LSD but stopped when she wanted to get pregnant, said, 'It was a time when I wanted to pay attention to my body, not escape it. Besides, I couldn't take it after the baby was born and still hear it when it cries.'

༄

Phencyclidine

Street names for this chemical change rapidly. It is also called PCP, angel dust and crystal. It can remain in a user's body for up to a year after use because it binds to fat cells. Studies in animals found ten times the amount of the drug in the piglet as in the pig, and those piglets, when born, did behave differently than others who were not exposed. No studies have linked phencyclidine use in women with a higher rate of abnormality in their babies, but babies exposed to phencyclidine are often stiffer and more agitated than normal babies at birth. Long-term effects are unknown because the relevant studies have not been done.

ॐ

Solvents and glue

Inhaled solvents reduce oxygen levels and easily cross the placenta. The effect of solvent abuse in pregnancy has been little studied but it seems that babies born to mothers who are solvent abusers have higher rates of kidney and bladder abnormalities than one would otherwise expect.

ॐ

Our attitudes to drug-taking in pregnancy

Babies cannot choose for themselves and most people feel deeply uncomfortable about drug taking and pregnancy. But I am also worried about legal moves to do something about the problem. In Britain, in 1986, the House of Lords upheld a care order for a child born to a mother who admitted heroin addiction. The courts said that she should not be allowed to care for her child and based this judgement solely on the damage done before the baby was born, damage which studies now show can be ameliorated with time and effort. She was not given that chance.

Everything I know about motherhood seems incompatible with what I read about addiction. All of us who have taken on the job know that being a mother means disregarding your own needs much of the time and focusing on what the baby needs. But I still find that court decision worrying and I feel that she should have had the help and support to give it a try. To do otherwise sets a disturbing legal precedent. Could this be the start of a slippery slope?

The 'slippery slope'

There has never been a shortage of people who order pregnant women to do this or avoid that. In the 1980s, judges in several countries showed that they were willing to consider enforcing such edicts. Some have already done so without, it seems, thinking about the consequences for other women. Here are questions I'd wish to put to them:

- If one woman was denied her baby because of damage by heroin, why not deny others because they smoke too much, or even drink too much?

- If you can rule after the fact, what is to stop judges confining women in pregnancy to ensure they avoid or consume drugs as ordered? This may sound far fetched but an American judge did order that a woman with no evidence of mental illness be kept in a secure hospital for the last two months of her pregnancy because he decided she was not caring for her unborn child properly. Half the doctors who run training programmes for American obstetricians, when asked, thought a woman should be confined against her will if she was behaving in ways that the doctor felt were dangerous to her unborn baby. Even if the place women are kept is the most comfortable hotel in the world, to confine them against their will denies a woman her own human rights.

- How can you be sure you know which women might be harming their unborn babies? The same survey of senior American doctors found that one quarter wanted 'state surveillance' in the last 12 weeks of pregnancy to protect fetuses. Also in the USA, criminal prosecutions have been launched against pregnant drug addicts, including for manslaughter and child abuse. In April 1991 a woman in Florida was successfully prosecuted for delivering cocaine to her unborn child, and a survey of American college students recently found that many would be willing to imprison women for using cocaine, alcohol and tobacco during pregnancy. Women who abuse drugs already shy away from antenatal care, how long would it be before they stopped going to hospital to deliver? Would society then need a prenatal police force to round them up? The doctors do not say so but these moves are part and parcel of their suggested 'surveillance'.

- If a woman can be punished for not behaving as a doctor would wish, does that mean that a doctor no longer gives advice but issues orders that can be enforced? That was the argument put forward by the prosecution who charged a woman in California with manslaughter after her newborn son died. The prosecution said she disregarded her doctor's advice that she should (among other things) stop taking amphetamines. A long and painful trial ensued before the charges were dropped. This attitude changes the relationship between a woman and her doctor completely. No longer will it be one based on mutual co-operation, but on coercion.

Mothers' rights and babies' rights

All these issues arise from the fact that before a baby is born, you cannot treat the baby in isolation. It's true that medical science provides more and more ways of inspecting, treating and manipulating the baby inside the uterus. Many doctors now regard the baby as their patient, some see the mother as a frustrating wall of flesh keeping the baby at bay. One doctor describes the unborn baby as 'the little aquanaut ... in intrauterine exile from the human community'. Yet none of these new and exciting treatments can be done except via the mother. When the mother refuses to treat the 'patient' – her unborn child – as the doctor wishes, the only option may seem to be to resort to the court.

Of course courts have the duty to decide who is and who is not fit to act as a parent for a particular child. They do this all the time and it is a proper function for them to do so. But the same cannot be said for a baby before it is born. More and more judges are asked to override a pregnant woman's wishes or to force her to act against her will. Many are only too willing to comply as the cases cited above show. It is now commonplace for American courts to be asked to intervene if a doctor deems it unsafe for a woman to give birth vaginally yet she refuses a Caesarean. Judges, unaware of how controversial

171

these matters are and how much doctors differ in what they consider 'safe', have ordered Caesareans in more than 24 cases. In a few the woman has given birth normally and without problems, before the order could be put into effect.

British courts have also intervened in decisions about a baby's welfare before birth, but they are much more reluctant to do so. Even so, civil libertarians follow these moves with concern. They point out that restrictions on the mother's freedoms, in order to safeguard the baby's, are not only unenforceable in many cases, they are contrary to the best outcome for the vast majority of babies. Babies in general will not benefit if you incarcerate a few mothers, if you force mothers to avoid or consume drugs and if you punish mothers if they do not. That diminishes the status and responsibility that society accords to all mothers because it treats them as incubators, not people. Many argue that since enforcement is only ever evoked against women who are poor, unsupported and outside the mainstream, we could use our energies more effectively by helping and supporting these few, rather than by creating a climate of opinion that undermines all women.

Nothing more effective than education, persuasion and support will help the babies whose mothers abuse them before birth. Going beyond education, persuasion and support in an effort to help *all* babies, will change every other woman's relationship with her own children for the worse.

LABOUR

Decisions About Drugs in Labour

Making the decision

This section explores drug decisions you could be called upon to make in labour. It will cover:

- drugs used to start labour artificially
- drugs used to speed labour up
- drugs used to relieve pain in labour
- drugs used to deliver the placenta
- drugs given routinely to the baby at birth.

Many drugs given to labouring women are not included in this list and, of course, any drug you are offered is a candidate for discussion and decision. You have the right to ask for more information, to take time to make up your mind and to discuss the matter with other people. You do not lose that right by being in labour. But in reality, parents deliberate about relatively few of the dozens of drugs that they *might* encounter while giving birth. The drugs that do get considered are the ones:

- that parents themselves consider important
- that can be predicted in advance
- that are not offered in an emergency
- and that involve real choices between well-supported alternatives.

Because you may be making choices based on these criteria, too, it may help to look at each one in particular.

Importance

Parents choose where to invest energy and attention, and some drugs never rate much of either. Take the case for and against taking an antacid in labour. This is a routine offer in many hospitals, made in the hope (some would say the pious hope) that an antacid will make your stomach contents less acid. Then if you should need anaesthesia and then are sick, vomiting less acid stomach contents would be safer. The rationale behind the routine offer of an antacid rates discussion in the professional journals – is it a good idea? Does it work? – but parents are disinterested. Antacids are little bother and have no obvious ill effects. Much better, parents probably conclude, to save their energy and attention for issues that feel important. The drugs in this section have been those I have found parents consistently interested in for the last decade.

Predictability and planning ahead

In pregnancy, you have months to talk, reflect and gather information. Some drug decisions in labour are like that, too, because they are part of the labour package offered by most hospitals to most labouring women. A few drugs (such as the ones offered to women with chronic conditions) can be predicted well in advance. And one or two (like those used in inductions) are suggested days or even weeks before labour begins. Women usually consider time spent discussing controversial drugs they know they will be offered as time well spent.

Time to think calmly

You might be curious about drugs to stop bleeding, to stop premature labour and to treat pre-eclampsia. However, if and when you are offered drugs for any of these things, you will be in the middle of a serious emergency. Your own or your baby's life may well be in danger, and deciding about drugs in such circumstances will be very different from other decisions discussed in this book, so you have to prepare for them in a different way.

In an emergency, what you will need is *not* prior knowledge gleaned from a few paragraphs on the pros and cons of a particular drug. What you *do* need is a trustworthy obstetrician and a good hospital. You can best prepare for an emergency by using your time and energy in pregnancy to find a doctor and a hospital you can trust. Caregivers who inspire your trust and communicate well antenatally, will probably do the same in an emergency. If they do not measure up antenatally, the list on page 253 will suggest groups who will help you find some who do. When you are too frightened, preoccupied or ill to think clearly, you will be glad you found someone who will help you make good decisions.

Clear alternatives

Sometimes, one choice has a very strong case. Take, for example, the question of giving steroids to pregnant women who are about to give birth to a premature baby. After investigating many studies, researchers concluded that premature babies have significantly fewer breathing difficulties when their mothers take steroids. I have met very few women who would continue to deliberate after being given this information.

The drugs discussed in this section are controversial because in each instance, a strong case both for and against taking the drug can be made and mothers debate fiercely on the advantages and disadvantages. They have the time and space to consider the choices before labour starts. These cases seem appropriate candidates for planning ahead and that's what the rest of this section will cover.

৵

Communicating your decisions to others

It may take some time to consider all the issues raised in this section but eventually, you will decide what feels right for you and your baby. When you do, that is the time to share your thoughts with whoever will be caring for you in labour. Your wishes are more likely to be heard and put into practice if you write them down yourself and if you express them positively rather than negatively ('Ben and I have practised relaxation and breathing techniques to help us in labour and we wish to use them to cope with labour. We hope you will wait until we ask for drugs before offering them for pain' as opposed to 'No pethidine'). Include a clear indication that you are willing to reconsider these thoughts throughout the labour.

Make sure that your written thoughts are included in your personal records and that the person caring for you in labour is aware of their existence. You may already be putting your wishes into writing about other aspects of labour care. These statements are often called birth plans and they are encouraged by many antenatal teachers and some doctors and midwives. Other caregivers find the exercise threatening and unnecessary.

If you haven't thought about birth plans in general, drawing one up specifically for drugs may seem rather daunting. You might find the book *Freedom and Choice in Childbirth* by Sheila Kitzinger (Viking, 1987) helpful. It first discusses why a plan might be useful, what topics you might include, and how you could phrase your wishes. It also includes plans written by several women and then discusses how the plan matched up with what actually happened. You could also get in touch with a local antenatal teacher or childbirth group (see page 254 for addresses).

Just as you need to communicate with the medical people who will care for you, you also need to talk these matters over with anyone who plans to support you in labour. If your partner or friends are aware of your decisions, they can act as your advocate if and when you are too preoccupied to do so in labour. Of course, they will need to remain as flexible and willing to adapt prior thoughts to new realities as labour unfolds, as you will yourself.

By planning ahead and then communicating your thoughts and feelings to those around you both before and during labour, you increase the chances that you will look back on labour with satisfaction. After the birth plan of woman named Kathy in her book, Sheila Kitzinger comments on her actual labour, 'As it turned out, Kathy didn't get all the things she asked for in her birth plan, but the relationship with her caregivers was so good and the discussion so open that from her point of view the birth went exactly as she wished.' The next few chapters may stimulate many thoughts and feelings. If so, you will help yourself and your baby if you share them with the people who will be with you in labour.

✑ 16 ✑

Induction and Acceleration

Deciding to have an induction

An induction is a procedure designed to make your uterus contract before it does so spontaneously. Inductions have been controversial since the mid 1970s, when doctors grew ever more enthusiastic about starting labours off artificially. In some hospitals virtually all babies were induced and, in many, it was common for as many as 60 per cent of babies born to be induced. Then (as so often happens in obstetrics) studies showed that wholesale induction was not a good idea. A few women and a few babies have had their lives saved, or their chances for good health improved, by induction but they only benefited if it was needed in the first place.

Doctors now concentrate on ever more accurate ways of discovering which particular women, and which particular babies, will benefit from induction. Because there is no agreement on this point, some induce as few as 3 per cent of their patients; others as many as 35 per cent.

Your first decision, then, does not concern the issues of drugs directly, but whether or not to accept an induction, should one be recommended. You should simply trust your doctor's opinion and agree straightaway – many women do – but an induction can be stressful and painful; it has risks as well as benefits. Many women say they can cope better if they are satisfied that they *do* need one and that they have tried other ways to start labour without prescribed drugs.

༃

Active participation in the decision

A leaflet on induction, published by the National Childbirth Trust (the address is on page 254), suggests that you ask five questions when your doctor recommends induction: Why do I need it? How will it help me and my baby? What are the alternatives? What are the risks and side effects? How will induction be attempted? What will happen if labour is not induced?

You may or may not find it easy to discuss these matters with your doctor. A special appointment rather than a snatched conversation in a busy clinic (possibly when you are the only person in the room undressed!) might help. Try taking along a friend or partner, read a book like this or other pregnancy books to gather information, and ask for specific evidence that an induction is needed in your *particular* case for this *particular* baby. If you accept that an induction is needed, there will probably be a gap between the decision and the procedure itself. For many women, that gap allows them the chance to find out about other ways to get labour started. The drugs your doctor offers are only one of the choices you have available.

༃

Self-help remedies to ripen your cervix

All through pregnancy, your baby is held inside your uterus by a ring of muscle called the cervix. Though a few women need a stitch in the cervix to keep it shut, and a small percentage of babies are born prematurely, for the majority of women the cervix stays tightly shut until the baby is ready to be born. Once that moment arrives, the cervix must change from a muscle that keeps the baby *in* to one that lets the baby *out*. This process is known as 'ripening'. An unripe cervix is thick, tightly closed and hard to the touch – it feels rather like the end of your nose. A ripe cervix is softer, more pliable and ready to stretch open as contractions press the baby down on it – it feels like your earlobe.

Ripening is not necessarily a sign that labour is imminent. I remember one woman who waited two weeks between the time her midwife said her cervix was ripe and her first labour contraction. A ripe cervix is nevertheless a welcome sign. It means that when contractions *do* start, the cervix is likely to open smoothly and fairly quickly. Many self-help remedies are aimed at encouraging cervical ripening. These include:

- making love – Semen contains prostaglandins (see page 184).
- nipple stimulation – Gently rubbing and rolling either nipple (using two fingers or a warm cloth) causes the release of prolactin, a hormone that softens the cervix. Various studies have been done to discover when and how to use nipple stimulation. The most common recommendation is that a woman should wait until she knows she is overdue and then massage a nipple for three minutes in every five, for an hour, three times a day, for three days. When she feels a contraction that lasts over a minute, she should stop. In one study, 45 per cent of the women who stuck to this regime went into labour as opposed to only 6 per cent in the control group. Those who stimulated their nipples but did not trigger labour had cervixes which were undoubtedly more ripe.
- acupuncture – One practitioner claims two treatments a day for four days ripens the cervix, and many women tell stories of contractions starting soon after acupuncture treatment, if their labours are overdue. Whether this is coincidence or cause and effect is unclear.
- homeopathic remedies – Caulophyllum 200 as a single dose is commonly prescribed. If you decide to use homeopathic remedies you will need to consult an experienced practitioner for the right treatment for you. If you have difficulty finding one, the addresses on page 254 may help.

Self-help remedies to encourage contractions

These remedies will only work if the cervix is already ripe. Even then, most of them are only effective in some cases.

- bowel stimulation – A dose of castor oil, a suppository or an enema designed to irritate the lower bowel, will cause muscle spasms in the large intestine. Sometimes, bowel contractions stimulate uterine ones. However, unless labour was about to start anyway, bowel stimulants just give you cramps and a bad case of diarrhoea. If they do trigger labour, the spasms castor oil causes can make it harder to relax and cope with contractions. I have known women so keen to avoid other drugs that they have accepted this.

  Some midwives say the baby, too, is affected by castor oil and also empties his or her bowels. This is something care-givers worry about because the baby's stool (meconium) will stain the waters. Normally, when midwives see stained waters, they grow concerned that the baby might be short of oxygen. So they could become alarmed unnecessarily or overlook real fetal distress. There is also an increased risk, once the baby is born, that he or she might inhale some meconium and develop breathing difficulties.

- herbs – Some women use herbs in their lives and feel confi-dent that they will also prove helpful in labour. A few are specifically said to affect contractions. The ones usually suggested are *blue cohosh* (one herbalist, quoting the experi-ence of Australian aborigines, says the herb 'does not stimu-late premature labour but can effect a more rapid delivery if labour is imminent'. She reminds pregnant women not to use this herb until the last weeks of pregnancy); *pennyroyal* (a Canadian woman, reporting her own experience, said it caused very strong contractions. It is said to cause miscar-riage if used early in pregnancy); *cannabis* (women say they find the 'high' it causes makes relaxation more difficult. See page 163 for effects on the baby); *red raspberry leaf* (I often come across references to this herb. Most sources suggest two or three cups of tea a day, starting from about the twenty-eighth week of pregnancy as a general uterine tonic); *spikenard* (herbalists claim this shortens labour).

Herbs are drugs and they must be used with discretion and care, following the recommendation of an experienced practitioner. You can find one near you by consulting the associations listed on page 254.

꒳

Accepting medical help for induction

Once you have weighed up the evidence in favour of intervention, discussed the various methods that might be used to start your labour, and looked into ways you might give Nature a push, you could eventually find yourself facing the decision whether or not to accept prescribed drugs for induction. Like the self-help measures described above, prescribed drugs have two aims: to ripen the cervix (the drug of choice for this purpose is prostaglandin); then, to stimulate uterine contractions (the drug of choice is oxytocin). It appears that prostaglandins are more likely than oxytocin to result in a vaginal birth. These drugs do not act on the cervix alone, although there is insufficient evidence to draw conclusions about their effects on the baby, or about whether prostaglandins are more or less safe for a baby than oxytocin.

Prostaglandins (Prostin, PGEZ) for cervical ripening

In 1979, 17 per cent of all inductions in the UK were preceded by a prostaglandin pessary; by 1986, that number rose to 64 per cent and it continues to rise. The drug is not yet in general use in the USA.

If you are offered prostaglandin, it will probably be in the form of a pessary placed against your cervix in the evening.

(Oral prostaglandins have not shown particularly good results.) You then wait eight to 16 hours for the effects. 90 per cent of all women achieve a ripe cervix; many women (up to 60 per cent of first time mothers and 80 per cent of those having a second or subsequent baby) begin to feel contractions.

Both these effects are welcome benefits. If you need more drugs to induce contractions, your labour following a ripe cervix (rather than an unripe one) will be less painful, shorter, less likely to fail because contractions will not become established, less likely to end in Caesarean section, and less likely to cause bleeding after the birth. One benefit in particular – fewer Caesareans following the use of prostaglandin for cervical ripening – is a significant change from pre-prostaglandin inductions. Formerly between 21 per cent and 30 per cent of all inductions ended in Caesarean section, 3 per cent to 16 per cent do so after a pessary.

Because cervical ripening is seen as so beneficial, the 10 per cent of women who have not achieved it after one pessary may be given another. It is unclear whether or not this is helpful. Repeated doses can make the cervix sore and increase the risks of side-effects, and they are often no more successful than the first try. You may want to discover your own doctor's preference before the first pessary is given. Many obstetricians now recommend that, unless the evidence in favour of induction is very strong, the woman should go home and try again another day.

Of all the women who are given a pessary, only a minority will need further drugs to achieve strong, effective labour contractions. If you are one of them, you will be offered a synthetic hormone (Syntocinon) that mimics the oxytocin your own body would make in labour (see page 187).

The disadvantages of prostaglandin use

The major worry about using pessaries is the problem of over-stimulating the uterus (hyperstimulation). This happens in less than 1 per cent of all women and when it happens the uterus contracts strongly and holds the contraction for a long time. As little blood can flow in or out of the placenta, the baby is denied oxygen and often becomes distressed. Drugs can be given to counteract overstimulation and make the uterus relax and extra oxygen helps, too, but a few babies will need to be delivered immediately by Caesarean section. Doctors hope to develop a pessary that combines prostaglandins with a uterine relaxant so that ripening alone occurs. Until they do, the problem remains.

Other side-effects are rare and less serious. Two women in every 1000 given a prostaglandin pessary experience nausea, fever and diarrhoea. One author calls this level 'negligible' and no sources mention any long-term effects. The drug does pass to the baby but no sources mention direct effects on the baby. Of course, if hyperstimulation happens, the baby will be put at risk, though one doctor, reviewing the evidence, notes that most babies delivered by emergency Caesarean for this reason are fine once they are born. Women with Caesarean scars may also be at risk, albeit very slight, of ruptured uterus.

Having a prostaglandin pessary also changes how the rest of your labour will be managed. You will no longer be seen or treated as 'normal', even if no further induction drugs are required. Many doctors insist that a woman given a pessary should be monitored to detect overstimulation. This in turn makes the mother immobile, possibly more anxious, and probably more likely to need drugs for pain relief. The doctor may have to break the waters to place the monitor, increasing the risk of infection, and committing the woman to delivery within 24 hours to avoid infection. Once you are there on the labour ward, caregivers may become impatient for your baby's delivery and suggest augmentation (speeding up your labour).

No one denies the benefits of prostaglandins for women and babies who need to be induced. Some people worry that simply because a pessary seems so straightforward and non-invasive, it will be suggested to women who would not otherwise be candidates for induction. We will need more time to assess whether or not this proves to be the case. For the moment, prostaglandin seems an established part of most doctors' induction repertoire.

Oxytocin to start contractions

Women in spontaneous labour produce a hormone (oxytocin) which makes the uterus contract. In induced labour, a synthetic form of the hormone (Syntocinon) is given via an intravenous infusion to serve the same purpose. Some doctors give the drug continuously, gradually increasing the dose; others give it in bursts (for example, for one minute in every ten) because this resembles spontaneous labour. Most doctors use an automatic pump to deliver the drug, starting with a low dose and doubling it automatically every thirty or forty minutes to a pre-set limit, or until contractions are strong, regular and effective in opening the cervix. When that effect is achieved, the dose will probably be maintained at that level. It may take some time to discover the right dose for you.

When Syntocinon is used, your baby's heartrate will be constantly monitored to pick up any signs of distress. An internal monitor is less cumbersome and more reliable than one strapped to your abdomen. To put it on, a doctor or midwife will break the bag of waters and attach an electrode to the baby's scalp. You may also be connected to a pressure gauge to measure the strength of contractions.

The advantages and disadvantages of Syntocinon

Syntocinon is relatively easy to administer and caregivers are familiar with its effects. The biggest advantage, however, is simple – it makes an induction possible. Without it, you would only have the option of a Caesarean delivery if it was decided that your pregnancy should not continue. With it, 95 per cent of women will begin having contractions within a few hours and their cervixes will begin to open up to let the baby be born.

The drug does cross the placenta but no direct effects on the baby have been noted. One researcher, interested in the behaviour of infants following Syntocinon, found no behavioural abnormalities at birth, no abnormal development, no abnormal intelligence scores, and no difference in motor development when compared with other babies.

The disadvantages of oxytocin are more complex than the advantages. They include:

- immobility – Intravenous Syntocinon ties you to a drip and a machine, and makes finding comfortable positions a challenge. This is one reason why more induced women ask for pain relief compared to women in spontaneous labour. One woman said, 'I felt like a trussed chicken with all that equipment and was scared to move in case I jiggled something.' Others are less daunted and move from side to side, sitting on the side of the bed with their feet resting on a chair and even standing by the bedside.
- sudden onset of contractions – In spontaneous labour, contractions gradually increase in strength and frequency and over several hours, a woman can adjust psychologically to the idea that labour has begun. She can also discover ways to be comfortable and help herself. With Syntocinon, the first contraction can last a minute and it can be strong enough to require all a woman's attention and relaxation skills. The next may follow within three or four minutes (or even one or two as the drug is increased) and carry on like that throughout labour. Women say such contractions feel 'spiteful'. One said, 'I felt like the first one knocked me over and I never really got back in the swing of things.' You *can* be ready, with good preparation, good support, and prior warning, to cope with that first contraction … then the next … then the next … just as you would in spontaneous labour. However, the pattern of contractions may be another reason why women being induced are more likely to use drugs for pain relief.
- over stimulating the uterus – Too much Syntocinon will cause a uterus to contract very strongly, hold that contraction

for longer than a minute, and contract again within seconds. Women find this painful, frightening and exhausting. In very rare cases, a uterus weakened by a previous Caesarean scar or many prior births may begin to split from the strain. Babies, too, register their distress when too much Syntocinon is given, through changes in their heartrates. These changes are caused by too little blood reaching the placenta to supply their oxygen needs or too much pressure on them from the contraction itself. Ominous changes in heartrates can be improved by slowing the intravenous drip, giving the mother extra oxygen, or (if necessary) an emergency Caesarean section.

- more complications – Women having inductions have higher rates of forceps delivery, higher rates of epidural anaesthesia, double the risk of having a Caesarean section and more risk of bleeding after the placenta is delivered. Some of these complications may be due to the reasons the induction was suggested in the first place, but many studies have shown that the procedure itself is the prime cause of the increase.

- negative feelings about the experience – Often the liveliest bits of someone's labour story are the ones describing the hours just before labour started. Parents wonder, 'Could this be IT?' Induction isn't like that. Induced labours mean clinical surroundings and messing about with drips and pessaries. Even if parents are grateful for the help induction offers them or their baby, they will have lost the excitement of early labour. Some women also say that accepting an induction makes them feel passive.

- problems for the baby – A few problems which were formerly attributed to induction are now less of a worry. Induced babies do get more jaundice and doctors thought this was caused by the Syntocinon itself. Now, it is clear that babies become jaundiced because they are not yet mature enough to cope with all the changes after birth. When induction was used liberally, many 'unready' babies were born, and some were very premature indeed, because delivery dates had been miscalculated. Neonatal nurseries had to cope with babies who had difficulty breathing, and a few who died. This was one very strong argument against elective inductions (those with no medical justification). Now, with doctors less willing to induce without evidence of real need, surprise prematurity is no longer such a problem and the 2 per cent of induced babies who are premature are anticipated and treated promptly.

๛

Drugs to accelerate labour

You may be offered Syntocinon even if your labour is not induced. This procedure is called acceleration or augmentation. You can get some idea of how likely the offer will be by asking your own doctor about his or her thoughts on speeding up labours. Some doctors only do this where the mother or baby shows clear signs of difficulty. These could include ominous changes in the baby's heartrate, ketones in the mother's urine (a sign that her body is short of energy and starting to use fat stores) or signs of dehydration. Other doctors do not wait for such signs but see acceleration as a form of preventative medicine. By prompt intervention, they claim to keep problems at bay. Despite its widespread use, there is remarkably little evidence from controlled trials about the effectiveness of Syntocinon in expediting labour. Of three trials, only one showed shorter average duration, in the others Syntocinon was no better than walking around.

Arguments for augmentation

Doctors who use acceleration freely have a clear idea of how long a labour should last, how quickly a cervix should open, and how long a baby should take to move down the vagina and be born. By breaking your waters and putting up a Syntocinon drip, a doctor can tailor the labour you are actually having, to match the pattern he or she believes is safest for you and your baby.

Pro-acceleration doctors often cite the experience of the Dublin Maternity Hospital where obstetricians prescribe Syntocinon to all their patients once they are sure a woman is in labour. (Labour is defined as starting when the cervix has begun to open and contractions are strong enough to be painful.) Once a woman is in labour, Dublin doctors 'start the clock' and begin to turn up the Syntocinon. Women are promised that the labour usually lasts no more than eight hours and never more than 12, and that the same midwife will stay with her until her baby is born. Enough Syntocinon will be given to achieve delivery within the time allotted.

The best known consequence of this form of active intervention is a very low Caesarean rate – 5 per cent in Dublin, compared to a UK rate of around 17 per cent and an American rate of 25–30 per cent. Dublin doctors also say women managed this way ask for less pain relief and report higher levels of satisfaction. Other hospitals who have copied Dublin claim lower Caesarean rates too (though not always as low), as well as lower forceps rates and fewer babies who need resuscitation or special care because of long, tiring labours. The Dublin results give pro-augmentation doctors confidence that they are helping mothers by speeding up their labours.

Some women, too, are glad they accepted acceleration. They report they felt 'stuck' because the cervix was not opening, discouraged by contractions staying the same for many hours, or frustrated by contractions that simply died away when the time came to push the baby out. They were told clearly why acceleration was needed, what would happen and how long their labours might continue. They say that once the choice was between a Caesarean, letting things go on as they were or accepting a drip to speed things up, acceleration seemed a welcome choice.

Arguments against acceleration

The women just cited as welcoming acceleration were ones who were convinced they needed the intervention because of evidence gathered in their own labours. This is quite different from women who are offered acceleration before the need is clear, on the grounds that making contractions stronger, longer and closer together is a Good Idea.

Doctors and women who are reluctant to use acceleration point out that there are other ways of achieving healthy babies and normal deliveries, aside from more intervention and more drugs. Dublin doctors may extol their 5 per cent Caesarean rates but the same rates are achieved by the French doctor, Michel Odent, who believes in offering women the space, help and support they need to give birth in their own way, and in their own time. By doing so, women have the benefits of the Dublin approach without the hazards of Syntocinon.

In the trials mentioned earlier, when women's views have been sought, over half of them said they found augmentation procedures unpleasant and over 80 per cent thought it had increased the amount of pain felt.

Taking a more laidback approach means that women can benefit from the changes in their own labour patterns. It often happens that contractions slow when a woman goes to hospital or when shifts change. In each case, a pause lets the labouring woman adjust to new circumstances. Sometimes, contractions stop in the second stage, then restart in a stronger form after the pause. Sheila Kitzinger calls this the 'rest and be glad' phase, but it is often seen as the trigger for using Syntocinon, as though a labouring woman had an on/off switch. Syntocinon solves the 'problem' of start-stop labours only if it really is a problem.

Precipitate use of Syntocinon also denies the woman the chance to try and restart contractions on her own. Darkening the room, kissing a partner, taking a warm bath, walking about or stimulating their nipples can all help. One midwife friend describes standing outside the labour room door to ward off intruders while a couple climbed into bed together to see if some stroking and cuddling would help (it did!). But few would contemplate such self-help remedies once a drip is up and staff are coming in and out to check up on it. Finally, accelerated labours, like induced ones, can leave negative feelings about the procedure itself or the pain relief that these new, stronger contractions necessitated.

With good support, prior warning and a chance to talk things over, both before and after the procedure, most women can come to terms with what has happened. Establishing when normal diversity becomes dangerous abnormality is an art. None of this is to say that Syntocinon is not useful, but liberal or routine use may not be beneficial or necessary. You and your caregivers will need evidence, patience and time, to decide whether adding Syntocinon to your labour is a good idea.

17

Drugs for Pain Relief in Labour – Making the Choice

Many women only think about pain relief when they are in labour and the doctor or midwife says, 'Something for the pain, Mrs Brown?' Once asked, they accept or refuse without prior knowledge of the choices available, or the consequences of each choice. They cannot do anything else – thinking with contractions in full swing is beyond most of us. Then afterwards, women have different reactions to their on-the-spot choice. Many are satisfied and feel that they would do the same again, but others are surprised or disturbed by the consequences of their decision.

This chapter looks at how you might plan ahead for that moment of choice. It presumes you have already learned something about labour itself before you begin to consider how you might help yourself cope with the pain in labour. There are plenty of good ways to find out about labour. Books, classes, experienced friends and your doctor or midwife will help you to piece together a picture of what it can be like, before you tackle the specific issue of pain relief.

When you do go looking for information specifically about pain relief, you will find no shortage of people ready to offer facts and opinions. But you will hear wildly differing things. One person will say 'If you have any sense, you'll take everything you can get.' Another will claim that the best births are those where the woman uses no drugs for pain relief. Particular drugs, too, have their own fans ('Try gas and air, it's magic!') and enemies ('Forget gas and air, it doesn't do a thing').

Nearly everyone will want you to agree with their point of view, although, fortunately, few are as adamant as the sixteenth century Scot who condemned a woman named Euphemia McClean to be burned at the stake for receiving an unknown medicine for pain during childbirth. Doctors and midwives, too, are partisan. Many will believe having drugs for pain relief in labour either is or is not a Good Thing and will use the facts they share to get you to think the same. If you meet two who have reached opposite conclusions, you might feel very confused.

To be fair, most authorities strive hard to be unbiased and objective – they put forward the advantages and disadvantages (in greater or lesser detail) and then suggest you make up your mind. But that turns out to be difficult, too. You may find Drug X, on the evidence offered, makes perfectly good sense but you do not *want* to take it; Drug Y sounds grand but it is not available; and Drug Z, though it has lots of helpful effects on most women, carries one or two very rare but very dangerous risks. How do they balance up?

Some parents act as though they would arrive at some kind of final decision if they only investigated the problem of pain relief thoroughly enough. This is a fantasy. Because the eventual decision hinges on so many variables that you will never arrive at a certain answer before the moment of choice. However, you can prepare for the moment by trying to decide which drugs are more likely to suit you and which you are extremely reluctant to consider. Your own choice will depend on:

- the kind of labour you hope to have – The next section of this chapter will suggest how you might find out if you find it hard to describe what your 'ideal' labour would be.
- the labour you actually have – Parents sometimes find it hard to accept that each labour is different but, despite billions of repetitions, each one remains an untold story. You may reach conclusions about what *might* suit you in labour, but you may well need to modify your conclusions as your own baby's birth unfolds.

- the attitudes and opinions of those caring for you in labour –
  Deciding which drugs will probably suit you best when you
  are sitting quietly at home is one thing. Communicating
  that decision to someone you may never have met before, in
  labour, on *their* home ground in hospital, is quite another.
  It is not always difficult – lots of women communicate
  smoothly and happily with caregivers, but you cannot rely
  on a tolerant and supportive reaction to your ideas in an area
  where so many have firm opinions. Opposing views could
  turn choice into conflict and you will need to be ready for
  that possibility.

On the other hand, if your caregivers know what drugs you are
hoping to use or avoid, what information you already have
about the choices, and what you hope your labour will be like,
they can offer appropriate help and support. When this
happens, parents continue to feel involved and that they are
making choices right through labour. Even when things do
not go as the parents had hoped, staff and parents alike can
look back on the labour that did happen with satisfaction
(tinged with sadness, sometimes, for lost hopes). I remember
a second-time mother who had sour memories of her first
labour ('It was more like a factory than a hospital. They sort of
put you on the conveyor belt and did it their way. One even
said, "We do it this way at St. M ...'s"). This time, she and her
husband practised all sorts of positions and massage techniques, aiming for a labour without pain relief. As it turned
out, things did not go quite as planned.

> John's mother couldn't come at the last minute, so John
> rushed around delivering the children and I went by
> ambulance. Then the midwife we were meant to have
> wasn't on call, so a new one called Janet arrived. She said
> the baby was posterior* which explained why it hurt so
> much between contractions, which I hadn't had before.

* With the back of its head against the mother's tailbone, often a cause of severe back
pain.

I'd had 'No pethidine' put in my notes but when Janet suggested some a bit later, I agreed because John wasn't there yet and I thought it might take away some of the back pain, which it did. Having Janet right there the whole time, helping me, made me feel it was still my labour even though it didn't go as we had planned.

Doctors and midwives are not mind-readers. They can guess what you might want in labour and what pain relief might suit you, but they will do a better job of supporting you if you tell them clearly what you wish to happen. One of the best ways to do this is to put your views in writing, discuss them with the midwife, and then have the final version attached to your notes. If this is a new idea for you, the suggestions on writing a birth plan on page 178 might help you get started. Your plan, like your baby's birth, will reflect your personal views on drugs for pain relief in labour. The rest of this chapter suggests ways of crystallizing what those views might be.

⌇

Step One: Finding your own birth style

To many parents, the idea that birth comes in different styles, to suit different people, is a novel one. They have a very strong image that there is a right way to do it and see it as their job to find that right way (or at least avoid the wrong ones). It takes a while to convince them that there are as many ways of having a baby as there are of doing all kinds of other things, like buying a house or going on holiday. Decisions about pain relief come *after* decisions about the kind of birth they want to aim for. There are no guarantees of getting there, of course, but drugs for pain relief can make it easier or harder to achieve the birth you want.

Sometimes parents have not any idea where to start when they are asked a question like 'What kind of a labour and what kind of a birth do you hope you will have?' You might feel the same. One way to clarify your thinking is to consider how you feel about three important issues: labour pain; the experience of being in labour; and how you would want to behave in labour.

Feelings about labour pain

While most people, when asked, agree that pain is to be avoided if possible and removed if it occurs, they do not all agree that the same holds true for labour pain. For some, pain is pain, and they want none of it. 'You don't here people talking about Natural Dentistry' they say or 'You wouldn't have your appendix out without anaesthesia.' One woman, asked why she chose an epidural for her baby's birth, said, 'Why go through it? It's just a question of how much pain you can go through. What is the purpose?' In 1986, the newspaper columnist, Polly Toynbee, wrote in a national newspaper that women who are reluctant to use pain relief 'surround birth with a bunch of mystical claptrap'. She described childbirth as 'agony ... pointless, meaningless pain for which, like many "natural" but bad things, there is at last a cure'. Feeling this way, she simply could not understand how anyone would *not* want an epidural.

But there are women who, when offered this journalist's description of labour, do not recognize their own birth experiences. Some births may be like that, they admit, but not all of them. They believe that as long as labour follows its usual, steady, not-too-long path towards birth, pain will not become stronger than a woman's abilities to cope with it. What happens when you give birth and what happens when you break a leg are both *called* 'pain' merely because the English language is short of words. Like the Eskimos, with their 27 words for snow, some women do not want to lump all the powerful, strong feelings that come with labour under one heading and call them all bad. Nor do they want them automatically removed.

Since pain is subjective and only labouring women know what they feel, we have no alternative but to believe them when they say labour pain is different from other pains. Labour pain, unlike the pain of injury, is not a sign that something is wrong.

> It definitely hurt having Jo but it was so different from the miscarriage I had before her. Then, I was holding back and frightened, saying 'No, No' the whole time. But with Jo, I wanted it so I could go with it, and it hurt less.

Labour pain also has a purpose – the baby's birth, it has a pattern; it waxes and wanes, builds up over time and so on. Many women find the rhythm and predictability reassuring.

> When I started to panic, Mike counted me through the contractions. He kept saying 'Twenty seconds and it will stop. Fifteen seconds …' then they did. I think we did that for a long time.

> I remember, right before I started to push, that bit between contractions. I have never felt so limp, so glad to feel at peace.

Labour pain has a time limit.

> At one point I felt it would be like that forever. Before this, I had a job, went shopping, but now I'd just spend the rest of my life on this beanbag, groaning. Then the midwife said something about the baby being low down. I know it sounds strange but I really had forgotten why this was happening until she said that. Then I thought, Well, it won't be forever …

Even the 'labour is different' camp admit that labour pain can *become* like any other pain if labour becomes abnormal or grows stronger than a woman's resources for coping with it. For example, if the baby is lying with the back of his or her head pressed against the mother's sacrum (a posterior baby), a woman can have severe back pain which does not go away between contractions. If women are anxious and frightened in early labour, they produce chemicals that can make contractions unco-ordinated and ineffective and these coupled with their fear and tension, can be very painful. Sometimes the inside of a woman's pelvis is shaped in a way that makes it hard for a baby's head to winkle its way through. It can take many hours and many strong contractions to get the baby low enough to dilate the cervix completely when this happens.

Some women will have the stamina and energy to keep going in all these cases; others will welcome pain relief. But until massage and moving about and kissing a partner and listening to boppy music and whatever else they want to try to ease the pain are not enough, many women feel that the risks of pain relief and the changes drugs bring to labour are not worth the unnecessary benefit of pain relief.

How you feel about the pain you might experience in labour is up to you, but it will have a direct impact on the decisions you make about pain relief. Only you know how much the benefit of pain relief is worth to you.

Beliefs about the role of labour in your life

Most obstetric textbooks begin with statements like, 'The goal of modern obstetrics is a healthy baby and a healthy mother.' Labour, according to this point of view, has no intrinsic value as an event in itself but it is merely a means to an end – the baby's birth. This attitude leaves doctors and mothers alike sympathetic to anything that will smooth the transformation from one pregnant woman to one mother and her baby. I remember a woman who summed up her whole experience as 'Great once the baby was there. Before that, forget it. I have.'

An American study asked women why they chose or refused an epidural (one form of pain relief that has the potential of removing all sensations from the waist down). One woman who had an epidural was pleased with her labour experience.

The end result is the same. Why go through it? It doesn't feel like I missed out on anything. I don't think I could have made it more meaningful or important. It's just a question of how much pain you can go through. What's the purpose?

An answer comes back loud and strong from women who are reluctant to use drugs for pain in labour. They see the act of giving birth as an intense, important experience in a woman's life, one that pain relief inevitably spoils or alters. When a woman labours, free from pain relief (and well supported by those around her), she can discover things about herself; she can discover things about her partner, possibly making the bond between them even stronger. She can prepare for the baby's birth, ready to welcome new life. Feeling proud and strong is the best way to start any new relationship, especially one as challenging and important as the one with your own child.

When a woman experiences these powerful feelings, she is keen to tell others about it. The same American study on epidurals includes quotes from those who refused, reflecting on their labours:

It was the most exciting experience. It's the greatest high in life. Giving birth is the only thing only I can do with my body. I feel more self-assured that I can control myself.

It's such a neat experience. I want to have it all! I want to feel the head, that warm bottom sliding through and against my thigh. It's a miracle of birth. It is an energy investment into when the two of you meet for the first time.

One British woman agrees that drugs can lessen the experience.

When my baby was put in my arms, I knew we had been through an experience together that was beyond compare.

I know that moment has been described a hundred times before, but it really is too spiritual for a poet's words. The freedom, lightness, energy and joy I felt then has stayed with me since. I'm sure this wouldn't have been so without natural childbirth methods.

Professionals, too, can feel just as strongly that labour is a chance to learn and grow. I remember one midwife who regularly told the story of walking into a room where a 17-year-old girl in very early labour was shouting for 'The Shot!' Eight hours later, with help, encouragement and constant support, she gave birth without ever asking for it again. The midwife considers this one of her success stories ('That girl took a big step towards growing up that day') and many of her colleagues would agree.

You may feel the same or you may feel more in tune with the women opting for an epidural because she wanted a baby, not a labour experience to savour. No one can prove that no-drug labours produce better mothers or show that women who experience little or no sensations in labour finish up diminished human beings. Both are philosophical positions that reflect the holder's own way of looking at the world. They also reflect how much energy and effort a woman is willing to invest in her own labour if she chooses to rely on her own resources and the help of those around her. Doing it yourself or letting others smooth the way – whichever side feels more comfortable for you will probably influence what you decide.

Appropriate behaviour for labour

There is no doubt that labouring women do behave differently than those going about their ordinary lives. Without pain relief, women can be noisy, restless, demanding and sometimes irrational; with it they are much easier to accommodate on a busy labour ward and much nearer to their everyday selves. Many women and their caregivers do not want 'a fuss'. One mother explained her decision to have an epidural in this way, 'It was wonderful. I sat up, chatting all through, didn't feel a thing. The baby just popped out and I went home a few hours later.' Another, wondering if she might want drugs, said, 'I don't want to be writhing around the room, down on the floor. Not that.' Drugs do make women quieter.

Caregivers too don't want a fuss. I have been taken around a delivery suite by a midwife who boasted how quiet her unit is more than once ('Nobody hanging from the chandeliers here'). One hospital assured all women with an epidural that they could watch television up to the moment of birth. Drugs help women cope by helping them 'keep control'.

Other women are uncomfortable with the image of quiet, compliant women watching television. They want a much more active approach to labour. They, too, want 'control' but it means something different. They want to do and say anything they feel would help them give birth. Drugs, they know, will limit this freedom to be actively involved. I remember a woman 'high flier' who said:

Once I heard that pethidine numbs the brain, confines you to bed and can cause strange thoughts, I thought yuk, not my sort of thing! Like being drunk – I hate that. What if I had to make some big decision about the baby or something, what would I do then?

Another expressed the same need when she said,

When I get tense, a walk helps me. You couldn't do that with an epidural, could you, not if your legs don't work.

Though they make the opposite decisions, each group of women is aiming for continuity with their non-labouring selves, reasoning that what makes them comfortable outside labour will do the same when contractions start. How you want to conduct yourself in your labour having your baby is up to you – if there was ever a time that belonged to you, this is it. Use it as you choose but what you decide will have a direct impact on what decisions you make about pain relief.

⟡

Step Two: Sorting out what's available

Before you make up your mind about what drugs you might like, you need to find out what other choices are available. Out of the scores of possible ways you might soothe the pain of labour, only a few choices will involve drugs. One woman I know found a self-help remedy to match every letter of the alphabet (A is for acupuncture; B is for breathing; C is for cuddles and cushions ... S is for sharing, sunshine, socks and shouting). Dozens of women have told me how helpful the things a woman can do for herself are. They praise moaning, moving about, sitting under the shower, music, plus lots of other things you can find out about in a good antenatal class. Above all else, they mention how soothing it is to have someone they love there with them, sharing the experience.

Hospitals can also offer non-drug remedies. A few have acupuncturists; many offer transcutaneous nerve stimulation via a small machine that sends pulsed electric current through pads attached to your back. Some have baths big enough to hold you, your midwife and your partner. Many furnish rocking chairs so that women can soothe the pain with rhythmic swaying. You could 'collect' all the available remedies in a kind of mental kitbag for using if and when you might need them. If you put into your 'bag' only the few choices described in this book you would deny yourself the full range of options available.

You might also consider remedies that have helped women cope with labour pain but which are not available on prescription or at your local hospital. The most frequently mentioned are herbal and homeopathic remedies. Neither has been evaluated in the same way as the more widely-prescribed prescription drugs, and no one knows what effect mixing alternative and mainstream remedies might have, but women say that they have found both helpful.

The problem with including these drugs in a book like this is twofold. You need to use different criteria for judging their use and effectiveness. One cannot, on the one hand, criticize doctors who disregard research findings and prescribe the drug they *feel* will work and then accept the same testimony from herbalists or homeopaths. Herbalists, homeopaths, and the women themselves all testify that alternatives do help. You must judge for yourself how much faith to place in these claims and in the skills of a particular practitioner.

At the same time, doses and combinations need careful, individual calculation. Herbs can contain powerful chemicals capable of harm as well as help. Individual responses are said to vary from person to person. One herbalist, discussing raspberry leaf tea said, 'It can be as wrong as it can be right.' She says she has to know the patient in order to prescribe and that she would never recommend women to treat themselves. When she does prescribe herbs, they are not given for pain directly but to 'improve, nourish and support the uterus in its work to expel the baby'. The list of addresses on page 254 will suggest organizations that can put you in contact with a herbalist who may then recommend herbs for labour. As there is no consensus as to which herbs are beneficial, it is impossible to predict which may be recommended.

What is true for herbs is also true for homeopathy – individual care and carefully-chosen dosages are what matters. You will need to establish a relationship with your homeopath well before labour to get the best care for you. Because few studies are done on homeopathic medicine, it is impossible to say what interaction homeopathic and allopathic (prescription drugs) medicine might have.

Prescription drugs for pain

Prescription drugs are available in hospitals and some are also available for home births. The ones you are likely to come across are:

• injectable drugs like pethidine (also called Demerol in the US) and Meptid

- drugs you inhale such as Entenox (nitrous oxide and oxygen; also called 'gas and air')
- and regional anaesthetics of which the most common is the epidural*

You may also be offered tranquilizers to reduce anxiety. The phenothiazines (promethazine, propriomazine, chloropromazine) and henzodiazepines (diazepam, droperidal) are tranquilizers most commonly used in obstetrics. They can affect the baby's breathing or ability to feed until their effect wears off.

You will need to talk to mothers who have recently delivered to find out *how* these drugs are offered in your particular hospital. Are they suggested? Encouraged? Left in the cupboard until the mother asks? This is even more important when finding out about epidurals (see page 222). If you are told your hospital does them, that could mean anything. You do not want to find out in labour that this means that epidurals are on offer every Tuesday afternoon if you book in advance. You will need to plan your questions well after reading the next chapter's general information about epidurals. You could ask:

- Is there 24 hour anaesthetic cover so women can have an epidural if they wish in labour?
- How far along in labour will they agree to giving a woman an epidural?
- How long does it take (on average) between asking and securing one?
- Can more than one woman at a time have one?

And so on.

You may also want to find out about provisions for emergencies should anything go wrong. Studies show the best

---

* These few drugs and techniques need not, of course, be the final choices you have, but to find others, you may have to change hospitals or seek out a new doctor. Either move has been helpful to women who felt strongly that they needed a particular technique, drug or service not initially on offer.

safety records are found where skilled, experienced people put the epidurals in and then have the people and equipment ready for accidents. Who does the epidural? Who can he or she call on to help? How long does it take for help to arrive? It is quite unusual for a woman to ask such things, but many would argue that this, too, is part of assessing the risks and benefits of an epidural.

No matter how good your questions, you will never discover everything or find out exactly what will happen. One labouring woman who had expected an epidural to be available (should she need one) was told on admission that one anaesthetist had broken his leg that morning and the other one was in surgery. The story ends happily – she felt no need to ask for an epidural after all – but does emphasize the need for flexibility. Good spadework should cut down shocks but it will never eliminate surprises completely.

↜

Step Three: Considering the baby's needs, too

This chapter, so far, has focused on only half of the people involved in a decision about pain relief – the mothers. What about the baby? As you will see in the next chapter, drugs for pain relief do cross the placenta and most affect the baby in ways we can measure and predict. There are also indirect effects on the baby either by causing a change that is dangerous to the mother, or by making other procedures more likely which, in turn, carry risks. For example, an epidural could lower the mother's blood pressure, something that threatens her health if it goes too low, and in turn, this threatens the baby. An epidural could make a forceps delivery more likely and, since forceps are also risky, the risk is then cumulative.

Healthy, full-term babies seem to cope well with the side-effects of pain-relieving drugs presently in use. That has not always been so. Until about 1960, no one considered the effect on babies when they pumped their mothers full of drugs for the pain. Doctors presumed it was normal for babies to be born with what they called 'neurologic shock' and that this was part of a baby's adjustment to life. Only later did they realize that what they were seeing was not physiological, it was pharmacological. These babies were full of too many drugs in too large amounts.

Then the pendulum swung the other way. In the 1970s, natural childbirth advocates gained access to the media and enthusiastic support. Mothers were encouraged not to use drugs and told both they and their babies would benefit from this. One researcher, Yvonne Brackbill, gained worldwide coverage for her claims that giving a mother pethidine changed the baby in ways that could still be measured at seven. She agreed with a reporter who asked whether these children had been 'born with half a deck'. These claims enraged the scientific community who all questioned Brackbill's methods (and a few questioned her motives). No one has replicated her studies or supported her claims.

As is usual in childbirth, views change and moderate. Pain relief now is more cautiously and carefully prescribed and we have the means to measure the effect on babies, and, what's more important, we are interested in doing so. In the 1950s and 1960s nobody noticed that babies were people with needs and feelings.

What we have not discovered (and possibly never will) is what these changes mean in the long-term development of a baby. Some alarmists point to the fact that a baby's brain continues to grow and develop until the baby is about 18 months old. Any drug could act as a behavioural teratogen right up to that time, just as a drug in the early weeks of pregnancy could alter an organ developing in a fetus. But so far, this is speculation. Drugs can build up to levels which are high enough to cause changes in the baby (see Chapter 18). But so far, these changes are noticeable for only a few days and occasionally, a few weeks; they are ominous only for babies who are already at risk because they are premature, too small or dependent on a placenta that is not working well.

No drug effects are of serious concern in the long-term health of full-term, fit babies.

It is important to remember, when considering *drug* effects on babies, that all labours will have an effect, with or without drugs. By avoiding drugs, you do not avoid *effects*, you just change what they might be. Epidurals may bring risks but they also conserve the mother's energy and oxygen and increase the amount of blood that flows to the baby. They lessen powerful feelings of pain, fear and anxiety that come with some labours and as it takes effect, the woman feels calmer, she breathes more slowly and deeply, and her body produces significantly less adrenaline. Her blood vessels open, she takes in more oxygen and more oxygenated blood reaches the baby. As the muscles 'let go', her baby may move more easily down into her pelvis.

These beneficial effects can last beyond the labour itself. We all know mothers who found labour a shattering experience and a few who continue to feel resentment, anger or fear afterwards. I know of cases where this has marred the mother-baby relationship, sometimes for many weeks after the birth. Pain relief might have been no help but it might have made the difference to how the mother welcomed her baby.

What suits most babies best is a labour that suits their mothers and takes into account any special risks either might have. In general, if you choose the labour that is best for you and the drugs most likely to help you achieve that labour, your baby, too, will have the best start in life. The next chapter will help you discover the pros and cons of individual drugs, as you make up your mind.

❧ 18 ❧

Pain Relief in Labour – Weighing up the Drugs on Offer

From the dozens of drugs you might be offered, this chapter concentrates on the half-dozen most commonly prescribed for women in labour, for labour pain. Each will reduce pain to a greater or lesser extent. All will change the course of labour once they are introduced. Every drug described will cross the placenta and have a greater or lesser effect on the baby.

Parents who have had the chance to review the choices beforehand say they are glad they did because they make speedier decisions in labour, they have a better idea how their partner feels and they have the words and expertise to discuss the issues comfortably with medical people. You could keep these benefits in mind as you read because not all of it will be comfortable to consider. Some side-effects are dangerous, others merely unsettling. But parents who have prepared for the moment of choice tell me they are glad they did.

❧

Pethidine (Meperidine; Demerol)

Pethidine (meperidine; marketed as Demerol in the USA) is widely used to relieve pain, including pain in labour. It is a synthetic version of the drug, morphine, and, like tranquillizers, acts as a central nervous system depressant. When women take pethidine, their brains register less pain, they worry about it less and so they relax their skeletal muscles more easily. It used to be thought that pethidine also relaxed the uterus, but this is not so.

The percentage of women who use pethidine in labour will vary from hospital to hospital, depending on how the staff feel about the drug and the alternatives available. In all studies the rates are falling. One London hospital reported that whereas 90 per cent of women used the drug in labour in 1970, only 15 per cent used it in 1985 and this was due, they felt, to the increasing use of epidural anaesthesia. Another survey found that where mothers could choose an epidural, 10 per cent to 40 per cent used pethidine in labour, where they could not, 50 per cent to 60 per cent chose pethidine. In the USA there is also a trend towards using smaller doses of pethidine, prompted by concerns about its longer term effects on the baby.

Pethidine is usually given by intramuscular injection into the thigh. In theory, the dosage is calculated according to the mother's weight (one or 1.5 mg per kg). In practice, most units use standard amounts, ranging from 50 to 150 mgs and your hospital will have one dose they usually give. You can expect to feel the effects within 20 minutes, and they usually last between two and four hours. Sometimes, pethidine is given intravenously, either as a one-off dose or, more rarely, through a patient-controlled pump that allows the mother to top herself up when she feels she needs it, within pre-set limits. The dose given this way is smaller and the amount that mothers give themselves is usually less than the amount given by staff. With intravenous pethidine, the effects will be felt faster but they will last for a shorter time.

It is impossible to predict what effects an individual woman will experience. Some are positive, helping her cope better with contractions and pain. Others are disturbing or unhelpful. For example in one NCT survey 70 per cent of women asked said that they found pethidine to be an inadequate pain reliever. Women who liked pethidine report:

- some pain relief – Between 20 per cent and 40 per cent of women say they received effective pain relief, and about the same number again say it was some help. Women say they feel distant from the pain, less worried about it, and so it is less distressing.

  > It was like floating along on a little pink cloud and I can't wait to get back there again some time.

  > The only way I can describe it is to say it took the top off [contractions]. They were still painful but not *as* painful.

- easier relaxation – Women say it allows them to 'let go' – they breathe more calmly and produce fewer stress hormones. Hyperventilation and high levels of adrenaline can make it harder for the uterus to work smoothly and less likely that the baby will get all the oxygen it might otherwise receive. Better relaxation improves both problems.

  > I just dozed off for a few hours, caught my breath, then started up again.

  > Between contractions, I could relax completely whereas before the injection, I was waiting for the next one.

Unfortunately, some women report distressing and unhelpful side-effects from pethidine. These include:

- feeling sick and possibly vomiting – How many complain of this is unclear. One study found that it is 15 per cent, another put the number who actually vomited at 30 per cent. Other injections can be given to counteract nausea (usually a small dose of a tranquillizer like promethazine) but they increase the mother's drowsiness and the negative effects on the baby (see below).

  > The pain was bad enough but contractions *and* heaving up for what felt like hours – Tom says more like twenty

minutes – was a nightmare. The next day it was a toss-up as to which was worse, my sore stomach muscles or my stitches.

- feeling dizzy – This is probably caused by the drug lowering your blood pressure. It is one of the reasons why, after pethidine, women must stay in bed.
- feeling isolated and unable to communicate –

  It felt like I was up in the corner, looking down on myself. It was not a good feeling.

  People kept asking me questions. I knew what I wanted to say but couldn't say a word.

- feeling confused –

  I was tired anyway, having lost two nights' sleep, and after the injection I found myself dozing between contractions. Instead of being ready, I was awoken abruptly by the beginning of each one, tensed with fear and pain. I just gave up trying to do anything. It was disastrous.

- being unable to hold or welcome the baby – If the dose is large and the mother has had time to absorb the whole dose but *not* had time for her body to work the drug out of her system (say, about an hour after the injection), she may feel 'drunk' when the baby is born. Some women do become clear-headed but others are unwilling to risk holding the baby. Often they are in no mood to try and some have experienced problems with bonding and initiation of breast feeding.

  John had to hold her in the delivery room because I couldn't have lifted a finger to save my life.

  You ask what Patrick looked like when he was born? I haven't the slightest idea. I was fast asleep after two injections of pethidine. I'm told he didn't cry much.

Coping with the difficulties

There are ways to mitigate the negative effects of pethidine. You are doing one right now – finding out what *might* happen. Women who believe pethidine will take away all the pain and are disappointed when it does not, make it worse. Those with more reasonable expectations accept and welcome the help they get.

Another way to help is to ask whoever is with you in labour to warn you that a contraction is coming. If your companion puts a hand over your pubic bone, cradling the bottom of your 'bump', he or she will feel the contraction about five or ten seconds before it becomes strong enough to rouse you. A quick shake ('Here comes one!') may wake you enough to cope with a contraction in whatever way you find works, and then you have the confidence to return to a restful doze. Your companion may find it hard to shake someone who looks so comfortable, but he or she will soon see that this is more loving than allowing you to wake in confusion and pain at the peak of a contraction.

A partner can also help with the moments just after birth if you feel unsure or unsafe because of pethidine. You could ask your partner to lay the baby across your chest or beside you. That way, you can get acquainted no matter how woozy you feel.

Timing your request for pethidine

This is tricky and you will need help from an experienced midwife or doctor. You do not want to ask for it too early in labour because unless contractions are well established, they may lessen or even stop after pethidine. Giving in too early also increases the chances that you will need more pain relief later on. Two injections of pethidine will cause the drug to accumulate in the baby, leading to more marked side effects than are common after only one dose. Most units will give more than one dose but all would rather not. One midwife said:

If the woman is very frightened in early labour, I think cuddles and hot baths work better than pethidine at calming her down. Then, if she still needs pain relief, she might do better with an epidural. It all depends on how she is coping and how fast we think things will go.

On the other hand, having pethidine late in the late stage is also not a good idea. In theory, staff aim to give it to a mother no later than four hours before the baby's birth. When they get the timing right, the drug has time to work and the woman's body has time to clear it from her own system so she can co-operate with the midwife in the second stage and greet her baby. More importantly, the mother (more precisely, her liver) clears the drug from her baby's body, too. Here's how it works:

- Twenty minutes after the injection, high levels of the drug build up in the mother's blood and continue rising for the next hour or so. They spill across the placenta, quickly balancing the levels in baby and mother. Since the baby is about twenty times smaller than the mother, and the dose is calculated according to the *mother's* weight (not her baby's), this may mean very high drug levels for the baby.
- Minute by minute, the mother's liver breaks the drug down and removes it via the kidneys. The levels in her body fall after two hours or so.
- As the levels fall in the mother, the drug flows back from the baby, to be broken down by the mother.
- Four hours later, most of the drug and most of the compounds made by the liver in breaking the drug down are gone from the mother. A little remains in the baby but much less than the original dose. Given too close to birth, the mother won't have time to benefit and the baby will be born full of pethidine.

The best decisions are reached when parents and staff work out what to do together. This often happens. Most women say that pethidine was discussed with them, although others describe the staff arriving with fully-loaded syringes and then discussing it. A few cannot remember being asked (whether they were or not is another question).

If you have strong opinions one way or the other, it will help staff if they know about them at the start of labour. Some parents have found it helpful to ask the staff to wait until they (the parents) ask for pethidine rather than suggesting it themselves. Others have welcomed the experience and support of a midwife or doctor when the time came to decide.

> Just before I started to push, I begged Ian to do something about the pain. I told him I couldn't go on. He says I told him I was going home! When the midwife came in, did an internal and said I was eight cms, she said, 'Come on. You're almost there!' She sounded really excited. She told me I could do it – so I did!

The effects of pethidine on the baby

Pethidine causes several changes in babies before birth. It reduces variation in heartbeat, something usually welcomed as a sign of a baby who is coping well with labour. If a tiny blood sample from the baby's head is taken, it usually shows a fall in the amount of oxygen in the baby's blood after the injection. Babies move less, too.

None of these problems are ominous in a baby who is coping well with labour, but for a few who are already in trouble, it could be one more burden to overcome. Some doctors recommend other methods of pain relief for babies who have been identified as fragile.

The effects then continue after the baby is born, especially if the baby has a significant amount of pethidine in his or her system. These last for as long as it takes to clear the drug and its breakdown products from the baby's system, which can take several days (estimates range from two or three to six or seven days depending on the dose, timing and size of the baby). Parents are surprised when they hear that it takes so long to clear, but a baby's liver is too immature and inefficient to do the job any faster.

If your baby is born with high levels of pethidine in his or her blood, you may not notice any changes at all. On the other hand, the first effect you might notice could be your baby's lazy approach to breathing. Pethidine makes babies less keen to breathe for themselves at birth and if the dose is large enough, some do not bother trying. In one US study, one in four babies whose mothers had received a dose of 50mg of pethidine within 1–3 hours of delivery needed assistance to get them breathing properly. They can be given an antagonist (usually naloxone) that quickly reverses the lazy breathing effect. This is fairly common and staff are well used to dealing with it. One study found no difference between the babies given pethidine and naloxone and those who had pethidine and needed no antagonist. Once again, respiratory depression is no threat to healthy, full-term babies but can be a problem if the baby is premature or poorly. In these cases, doctors usually advise mothers to avoid the drug in labour.

The next thing you may notice is your 'post-pethidine' baby's reluctance to suck vigorously and make an effort to feed. For a few days they can be a challenge to breastfeed. They are not interested, hard to latch on properly, and once they do manage it their sucking is often ineffective. Sadly, some women do not realize these are temporary difficulties and they give up breast-feeding. Bottlefeeders, too, have their worries. Some wonder if their lazy baby will be harmed by lack of food. Others adapt quickly to the post-pethidine baby's relaxed approach to feeding and then, about Day Four, when the baby wakes up and starts to suck with vigour and enthusiasm, think *that* is cause for concern.

If you choose pethidine, you may have to remind yourself to be patient and calm if feeding does not go well for a few days. One woman said the most helpful thing was to remember television pictures taken after the Mexican earthquake in 1985. Ten days after the quake, newborn babies were lifted unharmed from the ruins of a hospital, none the worse for wear after so long without food or water. It kept her calm and kept her going until her baby was more alert.

Pethidine also changes how a baby behaves for a few days. You may or may not notice these changes because they are so subtle that even people who are used to newborn babies find them hard to spot. Until the drug clears, the babies are less keen to make eye contact, less willing to pay attention to sounds and sights around them, less keen to hold their arms and legs tucked in and they are drowsier than babies who didn't have the drug. Each of these are minor in themselves but they combine to make these babies harder to cuddle and comfort. Most parents keep on trying and, in a day or so, they find their efforts more successful. Sadly, some may have their shaky confidence diminished even further. Why reach out to a baby that seems so disinterested? This may be why, even long after the drug is gone, we can see differences in post-pethidine babies and in their relationship with their mothers.

Researchers who find longer-term effects (several can measure differences at six weeks) may be seeing learned behaviour, rather than changes to a baby's brain as some alarmists have claimed. No one can say there are no long-term effects but the evidence is not there to support those who worry about serious long-term consequences for babies. If you know that you may have a few tricky days, you can plan to spend time coaxing the baby to feed and look back at you. Your new baby will soon discover both are worth the effort.

Using pethidine well

Pethidine is regularly compared with other injectable pain relief drugs and it comes out at least as good and usually better. One doctor said, 'It may not be great but it's the best we've got to offer.' It works best when it is given:

- several hours before birth
- in moderate doses
- for moderate amounts of pain
- when the mother knows the possible side-effects
- if the mother has good support

• and if the parents are patient with the baby after birth

If you do not like the sound of pethidine or if you think that it will not help you have the birth you want, it may be encouraging to be reminded of one study which found that women rated the presence of a single, supportive person throughout labour as more effective. That is one option. Another is to choose a different method of pain relief that might suit you better.

ॐ

Meptid (Meptazinol)

You may be offered this injectable drug as an alternative to pethidine. Preliminary studies in 1983 suggested Meptid might be an improvement because a newborn baby is able to clear the drug from his or her body more quickly. Half of the drug disappears in 3.4 hours compared to 22.7 hours for pethidine. Six or eight studies since then have compared Meptid and pethidine but not one of them reflects this earlier optimism. Both drugs offer the same amount of pain relief, they have the same side-effects (although one found Meptid users vomited more often) and the same outcome for the babies. Meptid works slightly faster but for a shorter amount of time. One study concluded: 'The most striking findings were the poor quality pain relief experienced by both groups and the high incidence of side-effects.'

If your doctor uses Meptid, he or she may be able to offer you reasons for the preference. Most doctors, on principle, will stick with pethidine, a drug with a long track record, unless a newer one is a clear improvement.

ॐ

Inhalation anaesthetics

The various options

You might be offered any of a number of gases to breathe in, either during contractions or during particular procedures. Women often find inhalation anaesthesia helpful if they have their waters broken before labour starts, or when their stitches are being done after the baby is born. Particular doctors and individual hospitals have their favourite drug amongst the many options and you will have to ask to know what, if any, they will offer you.

By far the most common one is Entenox, a mixture of nitrous oxide and oxygen (it is usually made up of 50 per cent of each but sometimes it is offered in other combinations). It takes about ten seconds to begin to work and lasts about a minute after you stop breathing it in. The use of Entenox has been reduced in recent years, partly because it can cause nausea and vomiting in some women, and probably because of concerns about staff exposure to it.

Using Entenox well

Women who like Entenox say they like the floating, lightly-detached feeling that it gives. They admit that it does not remove all the pain but it does reduce it enough so they can continue to cope. For many women (especially those having their second or subsequent baby), Entenox helps them cope with the end of first stage when they say they most need help with the pain. By then, pethidine and epidurals are both poor choices. Most hospitals would not offer an epidural this late in labour because the baby could be born before it started working and the mother would get all the side-effects, without any of the benefits.

Because you are in charge of administering the gas and because it disappears from your system in about one minute, many women are willing to have a go. If they do not like it, they can stop but many find it helpful.

> It was brilliant. Four big breaths of gas and masses of back rubbing got us through the next twenty minutes until the magic words, 'You can push'.

If you use gas and air, several things will make it more likely that you will like the experience:

- a sponge or something to suck to wet your mouth
- holding the mask yourself rather than allowing anyone else to place it for you
- taking some time beforehand to learn how to use it.

Here is one way that works: *as soon as* the contraction starts, take three or four deep breaths of Entenox. Then drop the mask and cope with the contraction in any way you can – complaining, breathing slowly, rocking your hips, whatever.

Do not breathe in gas and air throughout the contraction. If you do, you will finish the contraction with a high enough drug level to cause you to doze off completely. Since the gap between contractions is usually very short, you will then be unaware of the next one. Just as the gas fades, the next contraction will be gaining strength and you wake in a panic and grab the mask again. By the time the gas starts to work, the contraction is gone but you are full of the drug again. Quite soon, this technique insures that you sleep peacefully between contractions, full of gas and air, and you get no benefit when the contraction is in full swing! Women who do this find they are confused, in pain and sorry they even tried.

Whether or not you use Entenox is (compared to decisions about pethidine or epidurals) a pretty straightforward matter. Women can try it, see if they like it and stop if they do not. It is generally considered to have little or no direct effect on the baby because it is quickly expelled from the mother's system.

Even if the baby is born with high levels in his or her system, the first few breaths will clear the drug.

✥

Regional anaesthesia

There are several ways of reducing painful sensations by injecting small quantities of anaesthetic where it will act directly on the nerves carrying pain messages. You may be offered any of the following:

Paracervical block

This technique is used in the first stage of labour when most of the pain a woman feels comes from her cervix stretching open to let the baby out of the uterus. By injecting anaesthetic around the cervix, it is possible to reduce or completely remove these 'stretching' pains. Paracervical blocks are widespread in the USA but they are not generally used in Britain because the technique has two serious drawbacks: it requires a skilled obstetrician to do it; and in 1 per cent or 2 per cent of cases, it causes the baby's heartbeat to slow down from around 140 beats to 60 or 70 beats per minute and causes many more to drop less dramatically. This does not seem to cause any long-term problems for healthy babies but a few who are less able to cope have died from paracervical blocks.

Epidural anaesthesia

By far the most widespread regional anaesthetic currently on offer to labouring women is an epidural (shorthand for lumbar epidural anaesthesia). It is estimated that epidural anaesthesia is used in up to a quarter of all labours in larger maternity units in the UK. This procedure is described in detail in most pregnancy books and it is fairly complicated. You may find it useful to see photographs of the process, to talk about it with others who have had it done, and to question hospital experts, to imagine clearly what is involved.

Here's a brief run-through:

- An anaesthetist inserts a needle between two vertebrae in your lower back, entering a space alongside your spinal column called the epidural space.
- Once in the epidural space, a soft, narrow tube is threaded through the needle into the space. Then the needle is withdrawn, leaving the tube in place.
- Through this tube, an anaesthetist injects a drug (often either bupivacaine or lignocaine) which numbs the nerves carrying sensations from about the waist down. The tube is left in place and more drug ('top-ups') can be given should the pain of contractions return.

In study after study, epidurals come out on top when considering which of the analgesics currently available to labouring women is most likely to give satisfactory pain relief. Epidurals are also considered least likely to have harmful or distressing side-effects for either mother or baby. However, although epidurals are offered as 'safe', there has been relatively little research into the possible risks attached, and not enough is known about the short and longer term effects on women and their babies. There is some evidence to suggest epidural anaesthesia can prolong the second stage of labour and increase the risks of forceps or Caesarean delivery, and growing evidence of longer term side effects in women including backache, headache and bladder problems. The majority of women who have had an epidural say they would choose one again, but they do not suit all women nor is it always an unmixed blessing for those who choose to have one, and the following sections describe some of the advantages and disadvantages in more detail.

The epidural package

When you say 'yes' to an epidural, you are choosing more than 'just a wee jab in the back' as the majority of Scottish women in one study summed up their knowledge of the procedure. To receive the benefit, you must take the whole epidural package. Compulsory extras include:

- breaking your waters – This has to be done to attach an electrode to your baby's head. Breaking the waters also removes the cushion of fluid between the baby's head and the cervix so that more pressure is placed on it (and, of course, the baby's head). Once the waters have gone, the baby is open to infection from the outside world and so it must be born soon afterwards.
- an internal monitor – This machine registers the baby's heart rate and records any changes that could mean that the baby is distressed by the epidural or the labour.
- a pressure monitor – This records the strength of contractions and alerts the staff should they become too strong.
- an intravenous drip – This is mandatory because an epidural can cause sudden drops in blood pressure that will require prompt attention. Most anaesthetists use a dilute salt solution (such as Ringer's Lactate) rather than one containing glucose. Careful watch will be kept on the amount of fluid used, so that the woman and her baby do not receive too much and become 'waterlogged'.

Several procedures become much more likely with an epidural. These include:

- a synthetic hormone (Syntocinon) to speed up labour – This is not always prescribed but in general, the feeling is that once the epidural is working, it makes sense to have the baby as soon as possible.
- a catheter into your bladder – Some women are able to empty their bladders without the usual sensations but most

need help until the anaesthetic wears off. This is another source of infection.

a forceps delivery – Because you are effectively paralysed from the waist down, having an epidural will change how you push the baby out. Different units will have different ways of handling the second (pushing) stage of labour with an epidural in place (see page 231). All doctors will try and keep forceps deliveries to a minimum because they carry risks to the baby and the mother. A baby can be bruised where the forceps were applied or occasionally, be temporarily unable to move one side of his or her face. Women who have had forceps deliveries sometimes say they felt little discomfort but others describe the experience as 'quick but very painful' or 'like being turned inside out'. They are often bruised and will always have an incision (episiotomy) to enlarge the vaginal opening.

As this list makes clear, the advantages and disadvantages of epidurals are inextricably linked. You can not have one without the other so we have to look at the two together. That's how they happen in labour.

Epidurals have three important benefits: pain relief, reduced stress, and a controlled delivery.

1 Pain relief

An epidural that is working properly does relieve pain. This is by far the most common reason given for having one. Women say that this is why they booked the epidural before labour started and why they wanted one in labour if they had the option of an epidural on demand. When researchers ask women to assess how well it works, the percentages vary. 75 per cent reported full pain relief in one study; 50 per cent of the women in another who chose to have one described their labour as 'pain-free'; 98 per cent in another study said the relief was 'good' or 'excellent'. These differences probably reflect how the question was asked, what the women expected would happen and variations in the technique itself. An epidural is also useful for the pain in the first day after a Caesarean if it was chosen for the birth. Though it decreases a woman's mobility, it does keep her comfortable, alert and awake to her surroundings and her new baby.

Statistics do not do justice to the powerful feelings of relief and gratitude women have for epidurals, particularly if they have them inserted during labour itself, rather than before contractions began. Sheila Kitzinger, in a 1987 booklet called *Some Women's Experiences of Epidurals*, describes women who received an effective epidural in labour as 'its best proponents'. When her correspondents described their experience, they used many evocative words: 'The pain relief an epidural gave was often "pure magic", "a blessing", "indescribable", "a miracle", "like a prayer answered" and "blissful".' One woman said:

Within a few minutes I was blissfully numb and it was MARVELLOUS. I just can't emphasize enough how wonderful it was to be free of pain and to be able to think clearly again.

Such vivid testimony encourages women and doctors alike to imagine that epidurals banish pain completely, yet it would be wrong to consider even an effective epidural as offering an experience where you feel nothing. In a study that attempts to measure labour pain, a Canadian researcher asked women to rate the pain they felt on a scale of 0–40. Before the epidural, the average pain score was 27.9; 30 minutes after the epidural, they rated the pain, on average, as 8.0. I do not know (even after the scoring has been explained) what a '27.9 pain' *is* but I cite the numbers anyway as a reminder that 8.0 is not the same as 0. These women felt less pain and one or two might have felt none, but the majority felt some even after the epidural was in place.

Sometimes inserting the epidural is difficult – 2 per cent of women in one study described it as 'very uncomfortable'. Half of the women who wrote of their experiences to Sheila

Kitzinger* said the procedure was painful. Most women I meet describe twinges when the catheter itself is inserted but they say that this is a fleeting experience. In the Kitzinger study, those who described their experience as painful were often those whose partners were asked to leave, those who required repeated attempts by the anaesthetist to insert the needle (3 per cent of epidural attempts are unsuccessful because they cannot insert the needle), and those urged to lie still for a long time in labour while the insertion was accomplished.

Another unpleasant aspect for many women is what happens immediately after the drug is injected. Many (25 per cent in one study; 50 per cent in another) feel very cold and have bouts of shivering. This is usually a transient feeling and only about 10 per cent of women found it 'very irritating' in one survey. There have been efforts to improve this record – warming the drug to room temperature helps significantly; so does injecting a small dose of pethidine into the epidural space. Self-help is good, too; you could pack some woolly socks and a hot water bottle just in case you need the extra comfort. Because the inside of your body stays warm, the baby is unaffected.

A third aspect that can cause distress is a fall in blood pressure when the epidural takes effect. If this happens, women feel dizzy, nauseous and sometimes frightened. To counteract the fall, the anaesthetist will have an intravenous drip already in place and will usually give about 500cc of sterile water and dilute body salts before the epidural is established. Seven per cent of the women in the Kitzinger study were disturbed by a sudden fall in blood pressure.

---

* The Kitzinger study is referred to several times in this section because it aims to discover how women *feel* about their epidurals rather than how doctors view the results. To gather the data, women were asked to write in about their own experiences. The resulting sample is small (900 women) and it does not represent a random cross section of all women. By asking women to write themselves, the sample is biased in favour of those who have negative feelings about epidurals because people have a stronger urge to tell how things went wrong than how they went well. Nevertheless, this is still an important study because it is one of the few investigations of the feelings and long-term effects women are left with after they are discharged from hospital.

Short-term pain relief versus total pain experienced Pain relief for contractions is a short-term benefit and a very significant one. But some experts suggest that a woman should look at the issue in wider terms, considering the total experience of giving birth. A 1988 research paper describes an experiment with the amount of drug injected: when first-time mothers were given less of the drug, they did feel the contraction more but they were less likely to have a forceps delivery. Since having a forceps delivery and then recovering from one can be acutely painful (bruising and stitches are the things women complain most vigorously about), the authors suggest that a bit *more* pain in labour may well lead to *less* over-all.

In the same vein, some women are offered a different mixture of drugs which, in 70 per cent of cases, allows the pain to be removed without causing weakness in your legs. Doctors call this the ambulatory epidural and in theory, it allows women to walk around (though in fact, standing about is more like it).

Women who have had ambulatory epidurals report slightly less pain relief but much higher levels of satisfaction with their labours and less backache. They are also probably less likely to have a Caesarean section as being upright allows the uterus to work better.

After the birth, women who have had epidurals seems to be more likely to suffer backache, numbness and headache than those who have used other anaesthetics. Longer term studies disagree as to whether these difficulties persist. Several show twice the rates of long term backache (17 per cent of those having an epidural vs 11 per cent amongst those who have not in one study and 18 per cent vs 10 per cent in another). Other researchers have found no link between backache and epidurals. Whatever the case, many midwives now argue that women need to be told about the possibility of long term backache when deciding whether or not to choose this form one in 1000 suffer temporary loss of feeling or use of parts of the body. The authors report that all were fine after 72 hours with no need for special treatment.

Ineffective pain relief Not all epidurals are effective although I well remember one keen anaesthetist who assured me that all epidurals have the *potential* of being effective if you could just shake the woman about so the drug sloshed in to all the corners of the epidural space. Unless the anaesthetic is evenly distributed, a woman may continue to feel the pain or to be left with pockets of feeling. Some have feeling on one side and not the other and between 5 per cent and 10 per cent of all women report this experience. One who did wrote:

> Everything was numb except this spot about the size of an egg in my right groin, which was agony. They tell you how to breathe for contractions but not how to cope with that.

Women who have been promised relief then do not get it describe feelings of betrayal, anger and panic. When anaes-thesia is ineffective, pain actually increases. The study citing pain on a scale from 0 to 40 (see above) reports the numbers rose by 10 per cent after an ineffective block. On the other hand, Kitzinger quotes a woman who welcomed the uneven effect of her epidural. She felt contractions in the upper part of her uterus but not the lower, so she could tell when they were coming and push the baby out. Most women who have to cope with such feelings say that what helped them through was the good support and sympathy of those around them, although they found it hard work to re-gather their energy and courage to keep going.

Despite all the reminders of what *might* prove difficult, the fact remains that epidurals usually do work. They do offer the hope of complete pain relief. But they are not a panacea or a guarantee that all will go well. Again and again, women are grateful that they were told what might happen because, generally, it did not. But when it did, they had only the problem itself to cope with, not their own shock and surprise as well.

2 Decreasing the stress of labour

Decreasing the physical work of labour Stress hormones like adrenaline, are part of what gives labouring women the energy, power and will to keep going. A moderate amount of stress hormones helps normal babies prepare for the changes necessary at the moment of birth (for example the circulation changes). However, stress hormones do have side-effects. In the mother, they cause narrower arteries and higher blood pressure; they allow less blood to reach the placenta. If they rise too high, contractions are less efficient, less oxygen reaches the baby, and breathing patterns that don't work properly, like hyperventilation, are more likely.

This can jeopardize the health of mothers and babies who are known to be at risk before labour starts. Women with cardiac or respiratory problems, diabetes, those with pre-eclampsia and, possibly, those who smoke heavily, are generally thought to do better with epidural anaesthesia. All these women need to restrict the surges of adrenaline that are normally helpful.

Babies, too, might benefit from an epidural. If there is a known risk before labour starts, doctors often recommend epidurals. The most common candidates are mothers expecting premature babies, babies who have grown poorly in pregnancy or those whose placentas may not be working well.

Wanting an undemanding labour Wanting peace and calm in labour can have nothing to do with physical ills. Some women choose an epidural to reduce emotional stress. I have known women who feel at the end of their tether because of personal problems, tiredness, lack of support, or poor relationships with caregivers. They want an epidural 'to cut the hassle'. They may wish things were otherwise but they can see no way to make them so. Sometimes, they can be helped to see other solutions for their dilemmas. Listening, rest, good support and practical help can help discouraged women try for the labour they want, not the one they are willing to settle for.

But at other times, a quiet, non-demanding labour is important for a particular woman's wellbeing. One woman, looking back, knew exactly why she had chosen an epidural:

> I'm not one of those women who love being pregnant, and I was chasing a toddler all day. I was tired and overdue and James had already decided he didn't want to be with me this time. Fair enough. When the doctor suggested an induction, I agreed and asked for an epidural, too. If I was going to be on my own and all wired up, I wanted all the help I could get. I don't regret that decision one bit, but I do think if I did it again, I'd ask a friend to come with me.

3 A controlled delivery

An epidural takes away the urge many women feel to push their baby out: this can be helpful. Sometimes, doctors want babies to be born slowly and carefully and they like being able to control the delivery. This is often the case with breech babies, premature babies and twins – forceps are common in all these births. To use them well, doctors want a mother who can relax, wait and not push.

Unfortunately, having no pushing urge is not always a boon. It is one of the main reasons for a significant increase in the number of forceps deliveries that accompany epidural anaesthesia. Doctors are constantly looking at ways to reduce the number of women needing forceps because the procedure has risks for mother and baby. The risks are small if the doctor is experienced and careful, but mothers can be bruised and sore for days, because episiotomies are generally quite large and some will bleed more than expected, most are sore for several days. If the baby is bruised, jaundice is more likely.

To avoid these unwelcome consequences doctors have tried waiting longer before asking the woman to bear down, using less anaesthetic, letting the anaesthetic wear off towards the end of the first stage so a woman may once again feel her contractions, and increasing the amount of hormone drip

(Syntocinon) they give to stimulate contractions. All help a bit but forceps are still more common after epidural anaesthesia. The percentage of women who have a forceps birth after an epidural varies widely. In some units, the rates are about double the rate for non-epidural births (around 25 per cent). Some have higher rates (around 40 per cent) but they also have higher rates for forceps anyway. Asking for the rate at your own hospital will be a better guide than more general information.

Serious complications

Injectable pain relief like pethidine is more likely to carry unpleasant side-effects than an epidural. However, serious complications (though rare), are more dangerous with epidural anaesthesia. A 1995 report of births between 1990 and 1991 in 79 hospitals in the UK showed a rate of one serious complication for every 1000 epidurals, excluding dural taps (see below). 106,000 epidurals were studied and complications ranged from the life threatening to much less critical matters such as being unable to empty your bladder. When you are considering whether or not to ask for an epidural, you will be trying to weigh up very rare but potentially life-threatening complications, on the one hand should you choose this kind of pain relief with the more common, often distressing effects of other drugs. This seems to me quite impossible so I have no suggestions on how you might do this. I simply offer the information in the hope that it will prove useful.

Dural tap Putting an epidural in is a skilled job because it requires the anaesthetist to find quite a small space (the epidural space) without accidentally entering a larger adjacent one which contains the spinal cord. If he or she goes too far, he will puncture the membranes (dura) around the spinal cord, which is why this is called a dural tap. The chances of an unintentional puncture are very low. One study of 3500 births recorded 21 unintentional punctures; another hospital reports the encouraging news that their rate dropped from 4.7 per cent to 1.8 per cent in eight years. A 1996 study concludes that the rate now is 1 per cent.

There are two reasons why anaesthetists work so hard to avoid a dural tap. The most serious thing that could happen after a dural tap is the anaesthetic might spread too far and effect a woman's ability to breathe. This is very rare (eight times in 500,000 epidurals in one survey) but is the reason for having full resuscitation equipment to hand. If the problem is spotted before the drug is injected (and the anaesthetist has a whole series of checks designed for this purpose), there may be no problem. However, in about a quarter of all dural punctures, spinal fluid leaks out and causes a severe headache. There are ways of helping a woman with a spinal headache, including injecting some of her own blood to replace lost fluid (blood patching). This is usually completely effective.

Neurological damage It is hard to help women understand how rare it is that an epidural leads to paralysis or permanent lack of feeling. There was one case in a survey covering 500,000 cases and this one tragedy was caused by the wrong solution being accidentally injected. But it does happen. I remember how angry I was with an anaesthetist who was confronted with a quite hysterical woman who wanted pain relief yet begged, 'Promise me I will walk again.' He did. He had no right to, instead he should have said that the chances were miniscule – about the same as the chance she would meet her favourite movie star on the bus to work tomorrow.

The effect of epidurals on the baby

If one of the rare but serious complications occur, the baby, too, will be harmed by the consequences as much as the mother. Both share that risk and both are dependent on the readiness of hospital staff to cope with emergencies. The baby will also have a slightly increased risk from the other procedures which are part of the epidural package. For example, breaking the waters increases the chance of infection; forceps could pinch the nerve on the side of the baby's face and cause temporary paralysis; an intravenous solution can sometimes change the body chemistry for the baby, adding more glucose to his or her system or flooding the baby with fluid; and a monitor is useful for detecting problems, but it also increases the chance of Caesarean section for a wrongly diagnosed heartrate pattern, something that is quite common when monitors are used. These things need not happen, but by opting for an epidural, they become part of the total risk the baby faces.

But there has been little research into the risks of epidural anaesthesia to the body. A few studies have shown problems with rapid breathing for a few hours after birth. Several studies also document the *benefits* to the baby of epidural anaesthesia in labours where the mother was previously producing very high levels of adrenaline. After the epidural, blood flow to the baby increased as did oxygen levels in the baby's blood. After the baby is born, researchers note changes similar to those found after pethidine (see page 216) but they are less marked. One study showed detectable changes in the first month and concluded they were probably caused by mothers acting differently with babies after an epidural. The changes were very small and disappeared after this time.

Epidurals and Caesarean birth

If women know their baby will be born by Caesarean, they have time to consider what kind of anaesthetic suits them best. Reasons for choosing epidural anaesthesia include:

• wanting to be aware and alert – This is the prime reason most parents give for opting for an epidural. They do feel the surgeon tugging and some say they are uncomfortable. One said, 'It felt like someone doing the washing up in my tummy' but she felt this was a small price to pay for seeing, greeting and nursing her newborn baby.

Not everyone agrees. The best reason for refusing an epidural Caesarean is because you *do not* want to be awake and aware. There will be plenty of time to get acquainted with your baby as you recover from the birth.

- wanting to avoid the extra risks of general anaesthesia – Safety statistics are unequivocal on this point: both general and epidural anaesthesia carry risks of permanent injury or even death. In both, the chances of serious, life-threatening complications are very, very small but the numbers for epidurals are smaller still.

- wanting to avoid the after-effects of general anaesthesia – Getting better after a Caesarean is hard work, no matter what anaesthesia you choose, but an epidural leaves women less groggy and more willing to move about. Several studies show post-epidural mothers are more likely to try breast-feeding and more likely to keep at it than those who had a general anaesthetic. Their breastmilk comes in quicker too.

You may not have the choice of an epidural if the Caesarean is an emergency or the hospital near you does not offer the choice. If you can choose, it could be one way you can make your Caesarean birth as much like the birth you would wish for as possible.

Pudendal block

If you do not have an epidural in place and need a forceps delivery, you will probably be offered a pudendal block. A pudendal block starts with an injection into the walls of the pelvis, numbing the nerves from the pelvic floor and vagina. It works within minutes and, once effective, it takes away much of the pain of a forceps birth, though few women who have experienced a forceps birth would agree with one sanguine obstetrician who writes, 'An easy and painless forceps birth is thus possible.' They still feel lots of things: pressure, strong pulling, discomfort from being up in stirrups and so on. However, most women are extremely grateful for the help offered by pudendal anaesthesia in reducing pain once they agree to a forceps delivery.

The effect on the baby will depend on how much drug reaches the placenta. With most forceps deliveries, the gap between injection and delivery is so short that only minute quantities do so. Procedures that last longer may cause changes similar to those described after epidurals (see page 234).

Local anaesthesia for an episiotomy

The most common regional anaesthetic is the injection given to numb the perinieum just before a cut (called a episiotomy) is made to widen the vaginal opening for birth. Should you have an episiotomy, it is unlikely that the injection will be discussed with you. Most women are far too busy giving birth to notice more than a brief stinging feeling when the anaesthetic goes in. In fact, pressure and stretching caused by the baby's head usually numbs the perinieum well before this anyway. Because the baby is born quickly, there is no time for the drug to cross the placenta.

Stitching up an episiotomy (or tear) is another matter because you will have time to notice what's going on and you will have a keen interest in being comfortable. You will probably have (and need) more anaesthetic. The goal to aim for is complete comfort while stitches are being done – this way you relax and whoever is stitching does a careful, steady job. Women who have insisted on having extra anaesthetic are glad they did so.

> I'd never seen the man before who came to stitch me and he was clearly in a hurry. He started in the minute he'd done the injection. Thank God Jeremy was there and told him to stop. Once the drug started to work it was fine.

♪

Reviewing your choice

After your baby is born, you may find it helpful to discuss with the staff and your supporters what actually happened. You may have questions to ask or other information to gather before you understand the full story. You may also want to think about how you feel about the pain relief you chose – not to blame yourself if things did not go as you wished but to understand why you made the choices you did and whether, should you ever need to again, you would do the same. It may take some time and many tellings of your labour story before you begin to fit the pieces together and begin to put what happened when your baby was born into your own life story.

Drugs in the Third Stage

Drugs to deliver the placenta

In many hospitals, the doctor or midwife injects a drug into the mother's vein or thigh muscle as her baby's shoulders are being born. This is so routine that often the mother is not told of the injection and is unaware one was given. In Britain, the drug in question is usually Syntometrine; it is given to expel the placenta and make the woman's uterus contract into a solid hard ball. In the US, intravenous oxytocin (Syntocinon) is usually the one chosen. These drugs work within minutes (or seconds if given intravenously). By using them, doctors hope to lessen the chances that a woman will bleed from the site where her baby's placenta was attached.

Bleeding after childbirth is every doctor's (and many women's) nightmare. Once the placenta is detached, it leaves torn blood vessels that used to supply the baby's needs for oxygen and nutrition but now place the mother at risk from haemorrhage. The uterine muscle fibres surrounding each blood vessel prevents this from happening because when they contract, women bleed very little from the placental site. When they do not, a woman may lose a great deal of blood, very quickly. Between 1986 and 1989, nine women died from postpartum haemorrhage in Britain. This is a tiny number out of 2½ million births but it is nevertheless a devastating event for those nine families.

What is unquestioned is the need to minimize the chances of postpartum haemorrhage. But what some women and some caregivers question is the assumption that managing the third stage with drugs is the best way to achieve this. What you will have to decide is how you want your own third stage managed. The choice is between two 'management packages': one method includes drugs for everyone; the other witholds them until the individual woman demonstrates she is in need of them. The first step to making a decision is to be clear what each management package includes.

⁓

The active management package

In 95 per cent of British hospitals, the standard procedure for delivering the placenta is this:

1 As the baby is born, an injection of Syntometrine (Syntocinon and ergometrine) is given in the woman's thigh.
2 Within 30 seconds of the baby's birth, the cord is clamped and cut (to stop overtransfusing the baby).
3 The midwife watches for signs that the placenta has detached itself from the uterine wall (usually with a minute or so).
4 Then she puts one hand over the woman's pubic bone, and pulls down on the cord. The placenta usually slips out.

The Syntocinon causes the womb to contract within 2–3 minutes and the ergometrine causes a further contraction within about 7 minutes. The idea is to deliver the placenta after the first contraction but before the ergometrine takes effect.

༂

The physiological package

When a midwife or doctor manages a third stage physiologically, her prime aim is not to interfere with the complex and interconnected processes which complete a normal labour. After a baby is born, three things must happen for all to be well:

1 The placenta must detach from the wall of the uterus, come down the vagina, and be expelled.
2 The uterus must contract strongly and shut off any open vessels to prevent bleeding.
3 The baby must start to breathe and blood must flow into the baby's lungs to pick up oxygen. (Before birth oxygen came from the placenta and the lungs had little blood supply.)

While these three events are happening, the midwife 'sits on her hands and keeps her eyes and ears wide open', as one told me. The midwife encourages the mother to be upright, watches for her next contraction, then suggests the mother bear down. The placenta usually slips out. With his approach the midwife should not interfere (no cord clamping, no pulling, no pressing on the uterus) and not hurry the process.

The advantages and disadvantages of physiological management

The strongest arguments in favour of physiological management are philosophical. Mothers and midwives choose this option to be consistent in their approach to birth and in their views about drug use. They argue that if a woman can give birth to a baby, surely her body is also able to give birth to a placenta. They also point out that in pregnancy and birth, it is best to do nothing until you clearly need to. When a woman bleeds, wait-and-see midwives quickly give Syntometrine but they cannot condone giving all women drugs for the few who may benefit. This has never proved helpful in any other instance in childbirth, so why do it in the third stage? Besides, routine Syntometrine is powerless to stop life-threatening postpartum haemorrhage. Those nine unfortunate women mentioned above had plenty of the drug yet tragedy happened.

There are practical benefits of physiological management too. These include:

- a much more relaxed atmosphere
- a chance for the baby to get all the blood it needs through the open, pulsating cord
- less rush to be sure the baby is breathing well
- no side effects from the Syntometrine injection
- and probably less chance of trapping the placenta inside because of the strong contractions caused by syntometrine.

The disadvantages of physiological management are also both philosophical and practical. Many midwives are untrained in this style of placental delivery and many doctors have never seen a physiological third stage. They are probably frightened to do nothing, impatient to deliver the placenta and unwilling to hang about waiting for what can be as long as an hour or two until the third stage is completed. Parents often have the same feelings.

However, these disadvantages are hardly the most important factors involved. What really matters is whether women managed physiologically bleed more or face a greater risk of catastrophic haemorrhage. We are not short of people who say physiological management is safe because lots of people have delivered thousands of placentas without drugs. But until 1988, there were no randomized control studies to test which method was more effective at limiting blood loss. In November 1988, the *British Medical Journal* published the results of a trial of 1500 women done in Bristol. It was designed to provide the evidence we need to answer questions

about safety and haemorrhage. Those who support physiological management say the Bristol trial failed to resolve the
argument. (The trial is discussed in more detail in the
following section.) They continue to believe that physiology
can be trusted until proven otherwise. If you choose this
option, you must believe this, too.

The advantages and disadvantages of active management

Active management suits midwives because it is quick, familiar
and it is believed to reduce the blood loss from the placental
site. This is certainly the conclusion of the Bristol trial. The
authors report that 17.9 per cent of the women managed
physiologically lost more than 500ccs of blood compared to
5.9 per cent in the actively-managed group. The researchers
concluded that actively managing the third stage with
Syntometrine was justified because it did reduce blood loss.

Advocates of a physiological third stage management criticize the trials' methods and conclusions. They say testing
physiological management in a hospital where midwives are
unconvinced of the benefits of the physiological option, and
inexperienced as to how to carry them out safely, is no test at
all. Unless midwives know what they are doing and believe in
the woman's ability to give birth, they will never safety deliver
a placenta without active interference.

Advocates of active management say the trial confirms their
belief that Syntometrine does prevent blood loss. Women who
lose more than 500ccs of blood can feel fine but for some, the
blood loss will mean days or weeks of feeling weak, faint and
generally awful, until their body makes up the loss. Many will
need iron pills and a few will need blood transfusions.

Less partisan observers say we still need a randomized
control trial to resolve the issue. Sadly, the chances of getting
one following this well-publicized attempt is very low indeed.

However active management does have disadvantages.

- *side effects* – Women given Syntometrine are more likely to experience raised blood pressure, nausea and headaches. A few women are allergic to the drug.
- *early cord clamping* – If Syntometrine is given, the cord needs to be clamped straightaway lest strong contractions pump too much blood from the placenta into the baby. Because the cord is quickly clamped, no extra blood flows into the baby to fill his or her newly-active lungs. In a few babies, this leads to breathing difficulties.
- *time pressure* – A midwife or doctor must remove the placenta within seven minutes or the clamping action of the drug risks trapping the placenta inside, making a general anaesthetic and then manual removal more likely.
- *undiagnosed twin* – Very rarely, giving Syntometrine traps a second baby that no one knew was there. In these days of widespread ultrasound scans, this is quite rare but it is very dangerous for the second baby.

༈

Making your choice safer

Whichever course you choose, three points will make your choice safer:

1 Take the whole 'package' as described above, rather than picking and choosing which parts to accept.
2 Find out what the person actually supervising you at the birth is comfortable with, and then re-consider your decision in that light.
3 Keep an open mind. Events in labour may make it safer to have a different management package than the one you choose prior to labour. You will need to keep listening to the advice of your caregivers to make a good decision.

ॐ

Vitamin K for newborn babies

Your baby may be given an injection of vitamin K soon after birth. In the USA, this is a standard practice in all hospitals. In Britain, some hospitals give vitamin K routinely; others decide which babies are candidates for the injection. You may not be told automatically whether or not your baby receives the injection.

The reason for giving the vitamin is to lessen the risk of bleeding in the first week or so of life. All babies are born with low levels of vitamin K because it is produced by micro-organisms living in the gut. As adults, we have our own vitamin K 'factory' but newborns are born with 'sterile' guts and so they must pick up the micro-organisms from those around them before they can get the process going. In the meantime, their blood clots much slower than normal and for this reason, doctors now give babies particularly at risk of bleeding, an injection of vitamin K. Babies born prematurely, those fully breastfed, those born by forceps delivery, those needing surgery and those receiving antibiotics are often given the vitamin. Mothers who take anticonvulsant or anti-coagulant drugs during pregnancy are also likely to have babies who need it. However, other doctors recommend treating all babies.

There are risks for the baby from an intramuscular injection. The wrong drug has been given (this is now much less likely if the injection is given in the nursery rather than the delivery room). Rarely, a baby's muscle has been damaged by the injection. Some doctors now give the drug orally to avoid these problems and, of course, to spare the baby some pain. You may want to discuss all these matters before labour starts and include your wishes in your birth plan.

Looking Back – Looking Forward

You will never know, looking back on the decisions you have made for yourself and your baby during pregnancy and childbirth, whether you made the right decisions. You will have to settle for knowing that they were the best choice for you both at the time, given the information you had available and the things you knew about yourself.

This notion of 'no right answer, just one that seems best' is an idea that you may find hard to accept. People coming new to parenthood act as though, 'Should I take drug X?' is like the question, 'What is the capital of Peru?' Sometimes, it is – you shouldn't take thalidomide, you should stop smoking. But most of the time, things are not so clear cut. Usually, the question is 'What is best for me and my baby?' and that may have many possible answers.

After a while, experienced parents become accustomed to uncertainty. One mother who I knew was writing this book told me how she spent nights worrying about an antibiotic she took when she was pregnant with her son. Finally, she said:

It's twelve years since Mark was born and I feel just like that sometimes even now. I still wonder what's best for him and worry that he's safe, worry I made the wrong choice ... The other day, the bus bringing them back from a school trip was an hour late and I think my blood pressure was 200 by the time it came, imagining all the things

245

that could go wrong. I hate it that I can't protect him from danger, or be sure he's safe ... but I can't.

Such feelings do not become any more comfortable over the years, but you do get used to them. It is part of a chronic illness called parenthood and most of us are very glad we caught it! I hope you will be, too.

Glossary

Words in **bold** appear elsewhere in this list of definitions.

acceleration – an intervention used when labour has already started. By putting up a hormone drip (Syntocinon), contractions can be made stronger, longer and closer together, Snagging a hole in the mem-branes that hold the fluid around the baby can also speed up labour, by making contractions more effective and bringing the baby's head directly down onto the cervix.

alphafetoprotein test (AFP) – a blood test done at about 16 weeks to measure the level of this protein. A higher than expected level can mean either the baby's brain has not developed properly or the possibility of a spinal defect like spina bifida.

amniocentesis – a procedure done to obtain a small amount of the fluid that surrounds and cushions the baby. To do this, a doctor puts a needle through the wall of the uterus and draws off some liquid. It is possible to detect chromosomal abnormalities, like Down's syndrome, and some central nervous system disorders, like spina bifida, by examining the fluid in a laboratory. Final results take about three weeks.

anaemia – a lack of the oxygen-carrying molecule, **haemoglobin**, in the red blood cells.

augmentation – see **acceleration**

behavioural teratogen – If a newborn baby appears normal but acts or reacts differently from other babies, something has effected that baby during birth. If the differences continue, scientists now presume that the baby's brain developed in ways we do not see in normal babies. For example, babies born addicted to heroin continue to behave abnormally for many months after birth. This is a relatively new concept and is much more difficult to study than **teratogens** that cause clear structural change.

carcinoma – one form of cancer.

catheter – a pliable tube into a body cavity such as the bladder.

chelating drugs – used to remove poisons from the baby.

confounding factor – a problem bedevilling statisticians and researchers. Before they can prove that drug A causes effect B, they have to show that some other (confounding) factor could not equally well have caused the observed result. Here is an example: one study showed a direct link between heavy drinking and premature birth; when it was repeated, no such link was found. The first study was done on women with very low incomes; the second one on middle-class women. What had looked like a link between alcohol and prematurity was actually a link between poverty and prematurity. The poverty was a **confounding factor**. See **control group**.

control group – a group of people similar to those being tested in every way believed significant except that they are not given the drug, treatment or activity being investigated. Control groups are often matched for age, sex, race, occupation, number of children etc – whatever the researchers believe might be a **confounding factor**.

control trial – a study or experiment that looks at two different groups of people: one is given the drug, treatment or activity and the other **control group** is not treated in this way. Control trials are the best way yet devised to find accurate, reliable data on which to base clinical practice. See **randomized control trials**.

cytomegalovirus – one of the herpes group of viruses. This is the most common congenital infection and most women are unaware of contracting the disease. About three babies in every 1000 are found to have the virus at birth but only 10 per cent of those babies will have permanent damage caused by the infection. The chances that a woman will acquire the infection during pregnancy and that that infection will damage her baby are low.

dose-response ratio – a clear relationship between how much or how often a drug is taken and the good effects, ill effects or side effects of the drug. If, as is the case with smoking, the more you consume, the more damage is seen, this is a strong dose-response ratio. If, as with drinking, there is no gradual increase in damage as the amount of drinking goes up but instead, a sudden increase once a very high level is reached, this is a weak dose-response ratio.

dural tap – an accidental penetration by the anaesthetist of the membrane surrounding the spinal column. When this happens, either drugs can inadvertently enter the spinal fluid or fluid can leak out, causing severe headache.

embryo – a developing baby up until about five weeks when the correct technical term becomes fetus (foetus).

epidural anaesthesia – a complicated procedure done by an anaesthetist whereby a soft tube is passed into the small space alongside your spinal column. The nerves leaving the epidural space are numbed with anaesthetic injected through the tube. A working epidural can eliminate all sensations from about the waist down.

episiotomy – a cut done with scissors by the doctor of midwife to widen the vaginal opening. A local anaesthetic may be given beforehand but because the tissues are well stretched, few woman feel the incision. You will need stitches afterwards.

fetoscope – a flexible cable carrying optical fibres that is inserted through a small incision in the uterus and allows a doctor to see the baby inside.

forceps – an instrument shaped rather like two flat spoons used to deliver the baby towards the end of the second (pushing) stage of labour. Forceps come in several shapes and the doctor will choose ones best suited to the situation. Using forceps well requires skill and experience. You will probably be given a local anaesthetic before they are used.

haemoglobin – the oxygen-carrying molecule found in red blood cells.

haemorrhage – a sudden loss of blood. After birth, if a woman loses more than 500ccs, this is called a postpartum haemorrhage. Most women will need no special treatment though some will need extra iron and a few will need a blood transfusion if the amount lost is large.

hormone – a chemical produced somewhere in the body in a specialized gland and then carried through the bloodstream to another organ where it changes how that second organ works.

hyperstimulation – an ominous reaction in the uterus. Signs of hyperstimulation are very strong contractions that last more than one minute or that recur after only a few seconds pause. This pattern is caused by too much of the hormones oxytocin or prostaglandin, either produced spontaneously by the woman herself or (more usually), given in synthetic form by a doctor. Hyperstimulation can endanger the baby by cutting off adequate oxygen supplies to the placenta and can, in rare instances, cause the uterine muscle fibres themselves to split.

hyperventilation – an unhelpful breathing pattern, usually caused by stress. When hyperventilating, you breathe in and out deeply and rapidly, blowing off carbon dioxide. Your blood soon becomes too acidic; your baby gets less oxygen; you feel dizzy and your hands and feet tingle. The cure is to breathe slowly and calmly. Some people cup their hands over their mouths and rebreathe their own carbon dioxide until they feel better.

induction – a medical intervention whereby labour contractions are started artificially before they would do so spontaneously.

jaundice – a common condition found in newborn babies where their skins and eyes turn yellow. Blood tests reveal a high level of the chemical billirubin. Billirubin is formed when blood cells are broken down and it is usually removed by the liver. As a baby's liver is immature, it cannot do this job efficiently and billirubin accumulates. This is usually no cause for concern. However, if levels rise higher than doctors consider safe, putting a baby under special lights will help the baby be rid of excess billirubin.

listeriosis – a bacterial infection caused by an organism widely prevalent in the environment. About one pregnant woman in 7000 will contract the illness, usually from food such as soft cheese or pâté. In 1988, 291 cases of listeriosis were reported, 115 amongst pregnant women: 26 babies either miscarried, died, or were born damaged by the disease.

lumbar epidural anaesthesia – see **epidural**.

meconium – the sticky, black substance first passed from a baby's bowel. Passing it after birth is a good sign that all is normal; passing it before birth, causing the waters to be stained green, may be a sign that the baby is short of oxygen. Special care will be taken when the baby is born to make sure he or she does not inhale any meconium with the first breath.

mega-vitamin therapy – a controversial treatment based on the belief that taking vitamins far in excess of the daily recommended amounts will help the body work better and stay healthier. Benefits have not been proven. Fat soluable vitamins can accumulate to toxic levels. Taking any single vitamin in excess can upset the use and storage of other vitamins.

placebo – an inert substance that appears the same as whatever drug is being tested but has no pharmaceutical action. If a trial includes a placebo, it is possible to tell more accurately whether or not the drug itself has caused the changes seen because the researcher can eliminate the 'placebo effect'. The 'placebo effect' is seen when symptoms improve simply because people participate in a trial or receive treatment, regardless of what that treatment is. This is quite common.

pessary – objects containing some kind of drug which are inserted into the vagina.

perinatal – mortality rate between 28 weeks gestation and up to the first week after birth.

physiological – an adjective much preferred to the more widely used 'natural'. A physiological labour is one where the woman's body is allowed to function as it was designed to do; her caregivers withhold interference until the need arises. This approach is the opposite of a 'managed labour' where the medical team uses drugs, technology and intervention to tailor labour to a pre-ordained pattern.

potentiator – a substance that triggers the expression of a trait or defect. In order to do this, the individual's own genetic make-up must have made the person vulnerable to this particular substance. Unless both are present, the defect will not occur.

prematurity – see **pre-term baby**.

pre-term baby – a baby born before 37 weeks of pregnancy. The earlier a baby is born before 'term' (usually defined as 40 weeks), the more likely that baby is to have problems. Some will need special care in an intensive care nursery. Babies as young as 23 and 24 weeks have survived.

prophylaxis – a treatment or intervention begun before a problem is evident in the hope that the problem itself will not arise. For example, all women used to be given iron pills in the hope that they would not become **anaemic**. The current trend is away from widespread prophylaxis in pregnancy to ever more accurate ways of spotting the women who show signs that they do indeed need help.

randomized control trial – (see **control trial**). More accurate results are possible if the way people are allotted to either the trial group or the **control group** is completely governed by chance. If researchers select which people go into which group, the sample becomes 'biased' and the results are more likely to be influenced by **con-founding variables.**

ripening – a process that describes changes in the cervix just before labour starts. An unripe cervix resists stretching; it feels like the end of your nose. A ripe cervix is soft, stretchy and easier to open; it feels like your earlobe. Ripening is caused by hormones which change the fibres of the cervix itself.

teratology – a science devoted to discovering which actions, substances, and diseases can interfere with the normal growth and development of a baby before birth, resulting in a congenital defect or problem. 'Congenital' means present at birth.

teratogen – any substance, action, or disease organism that is known to harm a developing baby. A teratogen can change how the baby develops, resulting in structural abnormalities like cleft palate or heart defects. It can also change how a baby behaves (see **behavioural teratogen**), probably reflecting a structural change too subtle for our present knowledge to detect.

toxoplasmosis – 50 per cent of British women have antibodies to the organism that causes toxoplasmosis in their blood by the age of 40 or so. The disease has few symptoms and is usually contracted through eating undercoooked meat or handling cat faeces. If a woman gets the disease for the first time in the early part of her pregnancy, there is some risk to her baby. A small number of infected babies are damaged. Women are advised not to change catlitter trays in pregnancy though, if the habit is long-standing, the chances of a first-time infection in pregnancy are low.

variable – a term used in statistics to describe factors that could influence the outcome of a study. For example, how old the woman is, how many children she has, when she took the drug and so forth are all variables which will effect how a particular drug worked for her and what risks, if any, it posed for her baby.

Useful Addresses

MATERNITY CARE ORGANIZATIONS AND INFORMATION SERVICES

These organizations would appreciate a self-addressed envelope with any request.

Association for Improvement in the Maternity Services (AIMS)
21 Iver Lane, Iver, Bucks SL0 9LH
tel: 01753 65 2781
Information, support and advice on all aspects of maternity care.

Foresight
The Old Vicarage, Church Lane,
Witley, Godalming,
Surrey GU8 5PN
tel: 0142 879 4500
List of publications on preconception available.

Health Education Authority Folic Acid Campaign
Health Information Service
tel: 0800 665 544

Maternity Alliance
45 Beech Street
London EC2P 2LX
tel: 0171 588 8582

Publications and leaflets
Miscarriage Association
18 Stonybrook Close,
West Bretton, Wakefield,
West Yorkshire WF4 4TP

MIDIRS
9 Elmdale Road
Clifton
Bristol BS8 1SL
tel: 0117 925 1791
Information services including comprehensive database and publications related to midwifery and pregnancy.

The National Childbirth Trust
Alexander House, Oldham Terrace,
London W3 6NH
tel: 0181 992 8637
National network of antenatal groups.

WellBeing Eating for Pregnancy Helpline
27 Sussex Place
London NW1 4 SP
Helpline: 0114 242 4084
WellBeing: 0171 262 5337
Advice and leaflets about a healthy diet in pregnancy.

Women's Health Resource and
Information Centre
52 Featherstone Street
London EC1Y 8RT
tel: 0171 251 6580
Resource and information centre,
publications and leaflets.

COMPLEMENTARY AND ALTERNATIVE MEDICAL PRACTITIONERS

All these organizations request a
self-addressed envelope with any
enquiry.

British Homeopathic Association
27a Devonshire Street, London
W1N 1RJ
tel: 0171 935 2163

Institute for the Study of Drug
Dependence
Waterbridge House
32 Loman Street
London SE1 0EE
tel: 0171 928 1211

Institute for Complementary
Medicine
15 Tavern Quay
London SE16
tel: 0171 237 5165

Natural Therapeutic and
Osteopathic Society and Register
63 Collingwood Road
Witham
Essex CM8 2EE

The British Acupuncture
Association and Register
34 Alderney Street
London SW1V 4EU
tel: 0171 834 1012
1.30- 5.00 pm

The General Council and Register
of Osteopaths
56 London Street
Reading
Berkshire RG1 4SQ
tel: 01734 576585

The National Institute of Medical
Herbalists Ltd
56 Longbrook Street
Exeter
Devon EX4 6AH
tel: 01392 426022

Society of Homeopaths
2a Bedford Place
Southampton, Hants SO1 2BY
tel: 01703 222364

Traditional Acupuncture Society
11 Grange Park, Stratford upon
Avon,
Warwickshire CV37 6XH

STATUTORY BODIES

Association of Community Health
Councils for England and Wales
30 Drayton Park, London N5 1PB
tel: 0171 609 8405
Community Health Councils have
the job of representing the
consumer. This overseeing body will
offer information or put you in
touch with your local CHC.

National Drug Information
Network
Access to this is through your GP or
hospital pharmacist. They have
question and answer facilities and
also specialist files on drugs in
pregnancy.

SPECIALIST SELF-HELP ORGANIZATIONS

Action on Smoking and Health
(ASH)
Devon House
12-15 Dartmouth Street
London SW1H 9BL
tel: 0171 935 3519

Birth Defects Foundation
Chelsea House
West Gate
London W5 1DR
tel: 0181 862 0198

British Diabetic Association
10 Queen Anne Street
London W1M 0BD
tel: 0171 323 1531
BDA Careline: 0171 636 6112

Drugs and Alcohol: Women's
Network
c/o GLASS
30-31 Great Sutton Street
London EC1V 0DX
tel: 0171 253 6221

MIND
Granta House
15-19 Broadway
London E15 4BQ
tel: 0181 519 2122
·MIND Infoline: 0181 522 1728
x 275 (London)
0345 660163 (outside London)
Leaflets and information including
briefings on anti-depressants, major
tranquillizers and lithium and
pregnancy.

Miscarriage Association
c/o Clayton Hospital
Northgate
Wakefield
West Yorkshire WF1 3JS
tel: 01924 200799
Leaflets and information.

National Asthma Campaign
Providence House
Providence Place
London N1 0NT
tel: 0171 226 2260

National Society for Epilepsy
Chalfont Centre for Epilepsy
Chalfont St Peter
Bucks SL9 0RJ
tel: 01494 873991

Parents with Disabilities Group
c/o Judy Vickery
13 Chelsham Road
Clapham, London SW4
Holds a register of those willing to
talk with others with similar
disabilities.

Positively Women
347-349 City Road
London EC1V 1LR
tel: 0171 713 0222
Provides information and support
services for HIV positive women.

SAFTA (Support After Fetal
Termination for Abnormality)
29-30 SOHO Square
London WV1 6JB

Toxoplasmosis Trust
61-71 Collier Street
London N1 9BE

TRANX
25a Masons Avenue
Wealdstone, Harrow
Middlesex HA3 5AH

AUSTRALIA

The Department of Health in each state produces brochures on maternal and perinatal care.

The Family Planning Association provides pregnancy counselling and an advice and referral service for women. For details of your local association contact:
Family Planning Federation of Australia Inc
Suite 3, 1st Floor, LUA Building, 39 Geils Court, Deakin
ACT 2600
PO Box 26, Deakin West 2600 (postal address)
tel: 062 85 1244

Acupuncture Association of Australia
5 Albion Street, Harris Park
NSW
tel: 02 633 9187

Australian Medical Faculty of Homeopathy
tel: 02 809 6703
For listing of medical homeopaths.

Maternity Alliance
PO Box 214, Brighton,
VIC 3186
tel: 03 596 2650

National Herbalists Association of Australia
Suite 305, 3 Smail Street, Broadway 2007
PO Box 61 Broadway 2007 (postal address)
tel: 02 211 6437

Alcohol and Drug Information Centres provide 24-hour counselling, assessment and referral services. See telephone directory for local details.

NEW ZEALAND

Asthma Foundation of NZ
P O Box 1459
Wellington
tel: (04) 499 4592
fax: (04) 499 4594

Birthright
PO Box 6302, Te Aro
Wellington
tel:/fax: (04) 385 0103

Diabetes New Zealand Inc
PO Box 54, Oamaru
tel: (03 434) 8110

NZ Family Planning Association
National Office
PO Box 11515
Wellington
tel: (04) 384 4349
fax: (04) 832 8356

Pregnancy Help
National Office, Box 3808
Wellington
tel: (04) 473 7885
fax: (04) 473 7991

CANADA

Bay Centre for Birth Control
60 Grosvenor
Toronto, Ontario
tel: (416) 351 3700

Canadian Mothercraft Society
32 Heath Street
Toronto M4U 1T3
tel: (416) 920 3515
infoline: (416) 961 3200
Planned Parenthood of Toronto
36b Prince Arthur Avenue
Toronto M5R 1AG
(416) 961 0113

Pregnancy Care Centre
280 Aheppard Avenue E
Toronto, Ontario
tel: (416) 229 2607

References and Further Reading

I have not listed the source of every study cited or every statement made in this book. Rather, I offer a list of books and articles I found particularly helpful or interesting. Each of these sources will also have an extensive bibliography should you wish more information.

Background texts

Prescriptions in Pregnancy ed P. Rubin (British Medical Journal Publications) 1987; *Drugs in Pregnancy* D. Hawkins (Churchill Livingstone) 1987; *Drugs in Pregnancy and Lactation* G. Briggs et al (Williams and Wilkins) 1986; *A Guide to Effective Care in Pregnancy and Childbirth* M. Enkin et al (Oxford University Press) 2nd edition 1995; books written for prescribing physicians.

Toxicologic and Pharmacologic Principles in Pediatrics S. Kacew et al (Hemisphere Publishing Corporation) 1988; *Prenatal and Perinatal Biology and Medicine* ed N. Kitchener et al (Harwood Academic Publishers) 1987; *Perinatal Pharmacology and Therapeutics* ed B. Mirkin (Academic Press) 1976; books written for research-oriented doctors.

The Poisoned Womb J. Elkington (Viking) 1985; a book for the general reader on the threats to egg, sperm, and embryo from drugs, chemicals, radiation and pollution. *The British Medical Association Guide to Medicines and Drugs* ed J. Henry (Dorling Kindersley) 1988; includes an A-to-Z listing of common drugs with specific recommendations for pregnancy. If you buy one general-purpose drug reference book, this is it.

Obstetrics: a Practical Manual R. Neuberg (Oxford University Press 1995; British National Formulary, regularly updated list of drug advice includes a section on pregnancy with a table of drugs to be avoided or used with caution in pregnancy – in section on books written for prescribing physicians.

'Drugs in Pregnancy' in *Problem Drugs* A Chetley (Health Action International) 1993; *Women and Pharmaceuticals* (Women's Health Action Foundation) 1995 – discusses issues of inappropriate prescribing and implications from a woman's perspective.

Teratogen registers

(In Britain Contact the nearest branch of the National Drug Information Network. Access to this via a hospital pharmacist or your own General Practitioner. The Network has a question and answer facility and maintains specialist files on drugs in pregnancy.

(In Britain) Try the California Teratogen Registry, UC San Diego Medical Center, Dept of Pediatrics It-814-B, 225 Dickinson St, San Diego, Ca. 92103

Chapter 1
Suffer the Little Children P. Knightley et al (Viking) 1979; *Thalidomide: the legal aftermath* H. Teff et al (Saxon House) 1976; for the full story on thalidomide.

Chapter 2
NEJM 1983 308:8 424-31 and 308:9 491-7; for causes and frequency of congenital abnormalities.
Birth Defects and Drugs in Pregnancy O. Heinonen et al (John Wright) 1982; statistical analysis of 50,000 mother-child pairs assessing the risk of particular drugs.
Am J Obs Gyn 1989 160:5 ptl 1190-4; for women's perception of drug risks in pregnancy.
Towards a Healthy Baby: Congenital Disorders and the New Genetics (Oxford University Press) 1992 – general reference.
In J Gyn Obs 1992 39 185-6; *J Clin Epidemiology* 1993 46:6 581-9 – on proportion of pregnant women who take prescription and non-prescription drugs during pregnancy.

Chapter 3
Any embryology text book will describe fetal development. You could also read 'Behavioural Teratology' in *Perinatal Epidemiology* ed M. Bracken (Oxford University Press) 1984; BMG 1986 298: 6 Dec 1485-8.

Chapter 4
Am J Nursing 1985 85:12 1319; *BJM* 1986 292:15 Feb 494; on the problem of being sued.
The Unborn Patient (Grune and Stratton) 1984; for a description of what can be done and legal and ethical issues arising from treating fetuses.

References and Further Reading

Psychosomatics 1986 27:8 580-4; *Nervous and Mental Disease* 1986 174:9 509-16; *Neurobehavioural Teratology* ed J. Yanai (Elsevier)1984; Acta Psychiat Scand 1980 62:315-30; for the effects of stress on pregnancy and babies.

Chapter 5

The Health Conspiracy J. Collier (Century Hutchinson) 1989; a book about the practices that hinder doctors and harm patients.

To Do No Harm R. Apfel et al (Yale University Press) 1984; *The Custom-made Child* H. Holmes et al (Humana Press), 1981; *Pills That Don't Work* S. Wolfe et al (Farrar Strass Giroux) 1980; for more information about DES.

Ann Intern Med 1995 122 778-8 – update on DES.

Pre-pregnancy Care: a manual for practice G. Chamberlain and J. Lumley (John Wiley and Sons) 1986; *Planning Ahead for Pregnancy* S. Cherry (Viking) 1987. *Am J Obs* Gyn 1984 149:8 811-4; *Br J Hosp Med* 37:4 320-3; for an overview of all aspects of preconceptual care.

Chapter 6

In addition to the books listed above, these have been particularly helpful: *Clin Obs Gyn* 1986 13:2 189; on the risks of clomiphene (Clomid).

Teratology 1988 38:5 51-8; Obstetrics: Normal and Problem Pregnancies S. Gabbe et al (Churchill Livingstone) 1986, p 249; for the effects of oral contraceptives on pregnancy.

Br J Obs Gyn 1989 96:2 188-91; *NEJM* 1986 314; 25 1644-5; for the effects of alcohol on sperm.

Additional general references: *Getting Fit for Pregnancy: A Guide to Health Before Pregnancy and thinking About a baby: A Man's Guide to Pre-pregnancy Health* (Maternity Alliance) 1996; *Planning a Baby? A Complete Guide to Preconceptual Care*, S Brewer (Optima) 1995; *Be Fit and Healthy*, B. Pickard (Miscarriage Association); *Nutrition in Pregnancy*, M. Sadler (British Nutritio Foundation) 1994.

New Scientist 1992 17 October, *BMJ* 1996 312 506; *J Urol* 1995 154: 1030-4 – on smoking effects on sperm.

Chapter 7

BJM 1986 293: 6549 759; *Prog Food Nutrition* Sci 1986 10: 205-236. *BMJ* 1985 291: 27 Jul 263-6; *Occ Health Nursing* 1984 32:9 469-73; *Clinics Obs Gyn* 1986 13:2 253-65; for the arguments in favour of a 'good' diet (see also the book by Chamberlain et al listed above).

Alternative Dietary Practices and Nutritional Abuses of Pregnancy (National Academy Press, Wash DC) 1982; *Toxicologic and Pharmacologic Principles in Pediatrics* S. Kacew et al (Hemisphere Publishing Corp) 1988; for the dangers of megavitamin therapy in pregnancy.

JAMA 1987 257:10 1292-7; *Lancet* 1985 9 Feb 319; *Critical Rev Toxicol* 1979 6:351-75; for the dangers of too much Vitamin A.

Lancet 1985 II:9 1046-7; *Sci Total Environ* 1985 42: 121-31; for the pros and cons of hair analysis.

Arch Diseases Childhood 1981 56: 911-8; *Lancet* 1983 7 May 1027-31; for the original studies of the benefits of folates.
Zinc in Human Biology ed C. Mills (Springer-Verlag) 1989; *Drugs Ther Bull* 1988 26:8; *Am J Clin Nut* 1987 46:5 763-71; *Br J Obs Gyn* 1985 92:9 873-4; on zinc supplements.
Biol Neonate 1988 54: 263-9; on fluoride.
Current Concepts Nut 1985 14: 76; on copper.
Improving Infant Health (Health Education Authority) 1994 – general information and overview.
Nutrition and Health 1993 9 81-97, 99-106; *J Public Health Med* 1991 13:2 64-8; *Lancet* 1993 341 938-41 – fetal nutrition and health problems in later life.
MRC Vitamin Study Research Group *Lancet* 1991 338:8760 131-7; *NEJM* 1992 327:26 1831-5; *JAMA* 1993 269:10 1257-61, 1292-3; *Am J Clin Nutrit* 1993 58 127-8; Department of Health Report from an Expert Advisory Group 1992; *BMJ* 1993 306:6893 1645-8; *Am J Clin Nutr* 1995 62 782-4; *Lancet* 1996 March 9 657-9; *New Scientist* 1993, July 17 24-5 – on evidence to show folic acid supplements reduce congenital abnormalities, and folate sources.
Am J Clin Nutr 1994 59: suppl- review of issues related to vitamin-mineral supplementation.
Am J Obs Gyn 1995 173:1 205-9; *J Nurse Midwifery* 1995 40:1 36-40; *BMJ* 1994 309:6947 79-82; *JAMA* 1993 270:23 2846-8; *BNF Nutrition Bull* 1995 20 4-6; *Drug and Therap Bull* 1994 32:4 30-1 – on way routine iron supplementation is not necessary for healthy well-nourished pregnant women.
JAMA 1995 274:6 suppl 463-8 – on zinc supplementation.
Am J Clin Nutr 1994 59: suppl; *Nutrition and Food Science* 1991 128 6-7; Department of Health, Chief Medical Officer – dangers of too much vitamin A.
Department of Health 1991 *Dietary Reference Values for Food Energy and Nutrients for the UK* no 141 (HMSO) – recommendations about vitamin D intake; *Toxicology and Applied Pharmacology* 1976 35 393-5 – vitamin C and teratology.
Nutr Revs 1992 50:8 233-6; *Br J Obs Gyn* 1994 101:9 753-8 – On early evidence that calcium supplements may reduce hypertension; *Am J Clin Nutr* 1995 62 49-57 – discusses lack of evidence for reduced sodium intake to prevent hypertension.

Chapter 8
In addition to the books listed on page 80, these have been particularly useful: *Br J Sexual Med* 1988 15:4 126-8; *BMJ* 1988 297:6659 1324-7; for iron supplements and anemia.
BMJ 1987 294:Jan 42-6; for information on antibiotic, antifungal, and antiprotozoan drugs in pregnancy.
Br J Anaesth 1987 59:4 449-53; *Child Psych Hum Dev* 1986 17:1 66-70; for effects of anaesthesia in pregnancy.

JAMA 1989 261:5 728-31; *BMJ* 3 Feb 1983 no. 6376 728-31; for malaria treatment and prophylaxis in pregnancy.

BMJ 1985 291: 5 Oct 918-9; *Lancet* 1984 July 28 p. 205; *Neurobehavioural Teratology* ed J. Yania (Elsevier Science Publishers)1984; *BMJ* 1981 283: 11 July 99-101; on the supposed risk of Debendox.

Refer to general texts and also:

Am J Obs Gyn 1995 172:2 525-9 – meta-analysis of research studies concluding metronidazole not harmful in pregnancy.

Contemporary Ob/Gyn 1996 41:2; *Toxoplasmosis Trust Update* 1994 10 6-8; *Current Obs Gyn* 1991 1:2 62-6 – for spiramycin to treat toxoplasmosis.

Mat Child Health 1994 19:7 212 – erythromycin for chlamydia.

Obs Gyn 1991 78:1 33-6 – on vitamin B_6 and nausea; *Obs Gyn* 1991 93-6 – on antihistamines and nausea; *Can J Public Health* 1995 Jan/Feb 86:1 – Bendectin and nausea; *Br J Midwifery* 1994 2:10 495-8; *Obs Gyn* 1992 80:5 852-4 and 1994 84:2 245-8 – on acupressure, acupuncture and hypnosis and nausea.

Chapter 9

In addition to the books listed on page 259, these have been useful:

BMJ 1989 299:2 Sep 581; on epilepsy.

A Guide to Effective Care in Pregnancy and Childbirth M. Enkin et al (Oxford University Press) 1989; *BMJ* 1985 290; 5 Jan 17-23; *BMJ* 1985 292: 1129; on the treatment of high blood pressure in pregnancy.

Maternal Child Health 1988 13:4 103-4; on diabetes in pregnancy.

Drug Therapeutic Bull 1987 255:1; Chest 1989 95:2 supp 156-60; on anticoagulants in pregnancy.

Eclampsia Trial Group Collaborative Report *Lancet* 345 1455-63; *NEJM* 1995 333:4 201-5 – on magnesium sulphate for eclampsia.

CLASP (Collaborative Low-dose Aspirin Study in Pregnancy) *Lancet* 1994 343 619-29; *Comtemp Revs Obs Gyn* 1993 5;1 30-8; *MIDIRS Midwifery Digest* 1993 3:3 294-5; *Am J Obs Gyn* 1993 168:4 1083; *Lancet* 1993 341:8842 412 – on aspirin for prevention of pre-eclampsia.

Pregnancy and Diabetes B Estridge and J. Davies (Thorsons) 1194; *Diabetes Discovered During Pregnancy* K. Campbell and P. McParland and *Pregnancy, Diabetes and You* (BDA) 1995 – diabetes and pregnancy.

NEJM 1994 271:11 807; *MMWR* August 5 1994 43 and July 7 1995 44; *J Acq Immune Def Synd* 1994 17:10 1034-9 – on ziduvidine for pregnant women with HIV.

Obs Gyn 1989 73:3 526-31; *Int J STDS AIDS* 1992 3 316-8 – on acyclovir for treatment of herpes.

BJM 1993 307:6902 492-5; *Drug and Therap Bull* 1994 32:7 49:51; *J Perinat Med* 1994 22:5 367-75; *Epilepsia* 1994 35: suppl 4 S19-S28; *Pregnancy and Child Care and Women and Epilepsy* (National Society for Epilepsy) – on epilepsy drugs during pregnancy; *Lancet* 1991 337:8753 1316-7; *NEJM* 1991 324:10 674-7; *Arch Dis Child* 1991 66:5 641-2 – on tetraogenicity of carbamazepine for epilepsy in pregnancy; *Med J Aust* 1994 160:2 56:7 – on folate for women taking anti-epileptic drugs.

Obs Gyn 1991 77:4 504-9 – on cleft palate and benzodiazepines; *J Child Psychol Psychiatr* 1993 34:3 295-305 – on effects of benzodiazepines on long term mental development.

Asthma and Pregnancy (National Asthma Campaign) 1993; *Am J Resp Crit Care Med* 1995 1070-74; *Prof Care of Mothers and Children* 1994 14:7 198; *Obs Gyn* 1993 82:6 1036-40 and 5:1 25-9 – general information and evidence that good control of asthma can ensure positive pregnancy outcome; *Chest* 1995 107:3 642-7 – theophylline and asthma control during pregnancy.

Am J Obs Gyn 1994 170:3 862-9; *Chest* 1992 102:4 385S-390S – on heparin and risks of osteoporosis.

Obs Gyn 1994 83:4 616-24 – on calcium channel blockers for hypertension.

Mental Health: Dealing with Depression (Women's Press) 1996 – discusses approaches to treating depression and alternatives to drugs; *JAMA* 1993 269:17 2246-8; *Women and Pharmaceuticals* – on Prozac.

BMJ 1989 299:2 Sep 581; on epilepsy.

Chapter 10
In addition to the books listed on page 259, you could consult:

Medicines: a Guide for Everybody P. Parish (Penguin) 1989; *BMJ* 1986 293: 13 Dec 1549-50; Obstetrics: Normal and Problem Pregnancies S. Grabbe et al (Churchill Livingstone) 1986; for more information on over-the-counter drugs.

Nursing Times 1988 84:37 20-1; for a discussion of the aspirin trial.

Br J Preventative Soc Med 1961 15:154-66 *Lancet* 1978 2:634; *Lancet* 1979 1:1403; for risks of fever in pregnancy.

Lancet March, 1982; *Cal Assoc Midwives Newsletter* Jan, 1985; for the benefits of ginger.

Am J Obs Gyn 157:5 1286-40; *Occ Health Nursing* 1984 32:9 469-73; for the effects of caffeine in pregnancy.

Drugs, Pregnancy and Childcare (ISDD) 1995; *Am J Public Health* 1992 82 85091; *JAMA* 1993 270:24 2973–2974 & 2940–3; *JAMA* 1993 269:5 593-7; *Am J Obs Gyn* 1991 164:4 1109-14 – for reviews of evidence and different views about the dangers of caffeine.

Chapter 11
Weiner's Herbal M. Weiner (Stern and Doubleday) 1980; *Herbs for Pregnancy and Childbirth* A. McIntyre (Sheldon Press) 1988; *Homeopathy – the family handybook* (Unwin)1987; for more information.

Drug Therapeutic Bull 24:25; *J Pediatr* 1988 Mar 112:3 433-6; *So Af Med J* 1987 71:431-3; *Nature* 1072 238:106-7; on the dangers of herbs in pregnancy.

J Nurse Midwifery 1987 Jul-Aug 32:4 260-2; on the usefulness of herbs in pregnancy.

Midwives Chron 1988 101:1205 185-7 and 101:1206 222-6; for the use of homeopathy in midwifery.

Complementary Therapies for Pregnancy and Childbirth D Tiran and S Mack (Balliere Tindall) 1995; *Homeopathic Medicines for Pregnancy and Childbirth* R Moskowitz (North Atlantic Books and Homeopathic Educational Services) 1992; *Your Natural Pregnancy: A Guide to Comp-lementary Therapy* A. Charlish (Boxtree) 1995 – for more information.

Chapter 12
Alcohol and the Fetus H. Rosett and L. Weiner (Oxford University Press) 1984; *Women, Drinking and Pregnancy* M. Plant (Tavistock Pub-lications 1984; 'Alcohol and Pregnancy' *ICEA Review* 1984 8:2; for a review of the dangers of drinking in pregnancy.
Am J Obs Gyn 1987 156:1 33-9; 'Fact Sheet: FAS' in Midwives Information Service no. 5 1987; *Pediatrics* 1987 80:3 309-14; *Alcohol* 1986 3: 269-72; on alcohol as a teratogen.
Br J Obs Gyn 1989 96:2 188-91; *BMJ* 1989 298:6676 795-801; *JAMA* 1986 255: 1 82-4; *Lancet*, 1983 1:26 Mar pp. 663-5; *NEJM* 308:9 491-7; on the negative effects of heavy drinking on pregnancy.
NEJM 1986 314:25 1644-5; for the effects of father's drinking.
Am J Obs Gyn 1989 160:4 863-70; on risk drinking and binges in pregnancy.
Obs Gyn 1987 69:4 594-7; *Br J Obs Gyn* 1988 95:3 243-7; on patterns of drinking and their effect on pregnancy.
Science 1981 214: 6 Nov 642-4; *Sunday Times* 30 April 1989; on the conse-quences of an absolute ban on alcohol.
Alcohol and Pregnancy (MIDIRS and NHS Centre for Reviews and Dissemination) 1996; *Drugs, Pregnancy and Childcare* (ISDD) 1995 – for an overview of the evidence and practical advice.
Alcoholism 1988 23:3 229-33; *Am J Pub Health* 1991 81 69-73; *Am J Pub Health* 1992 82 87-91 – on combined effects of alcohol and smoking, and caffeine.
Int J Epidemiology 1992 21:suppl 1; *Alcoholism* 25:213 287-91; Lancet 1993 341:8850 907-10; *Am J Public Health* 85:12 1654-61 – on effects of alcohol – on birthweight and longer term child development.
Br J Addiction 1991 86 1063-73; *Alcohol & Alcoholism* 1995 30:3 345-55; *Int J Epidemiology* 1992 21:4 suppl 1 S1-S87; *BMJ* 1991 303:6793 22-6 – for review of evidence that moderate drinking is not harmful; *Epidemiology* 1993 4:5 415-20 – for review of evidence for risks of occasional binge drinking.

Chapter 13
Am J Pub Health 1987 77:7 83-5; *J Royal Coll Gen Prac* April 1986; *Am J Obs Gyn* 1977 128: 494; *Am J Epidemiology* 1985 121:4-6; *BMJ* 1984 11 Feb 288: 424; for a review of the effects of smoking in pregnancy.
Banishing Tobacco W. Chandler Worldwatch paper 68, Worldwatch Institute, Washington DC 1986; *Lancet* August, 1986; *NEJM* 1986 315:25 1551; on the dangers of passive smoking.
Beating the Ladykillers B. Jacobsen (Pluto) 1986; *Health Visitor* 1989 62: 22-4; on women and smoking.

Principles for Evaluating Health Risks to Progeny with Exposure to Chemicals During Pregnancy Environmental Health Criteria series, (World Health Organisation, Geneva) 1984; 'Effects of smoking during pregnancy on the mother' *Lancet* 1986 1:8494 1350-2; *Lancet* 21 Mar, 1981 p. 627; for the effects of smoking around conception.

JAMA 1986 255: 82-4; on smoking and prematurity.

Int J Epidemiol 16:1 44-51; *Br J Obs Gyn* 1988 95:6 551-5; on smoking and low birth weight.

Am J Epidemiology 1975 100:6 423-52; on the increase in baby death from smoking.

Med J Aust 1988 148: April 381-4; on how pregnant women feel about their smoking.

Smoking and Pregnancy (Health Education Authority) 1994 – first section gives a good overview of current knowledge.

Smoking and Pregnancy: Tracking Surveys (HEA) 1993 – attitudes of pregnant women about dangers of smoking.

Paed Perinat Epidemiology 1995 9:4 381-90; *J Fam Practice* 195 40:4 385-94; *Pediatrics* 1992 90:6 905-8; *J Smoking Rel Dis* 1994 5: supp 113-8; *Am J Respir Crit Care Med* 1995 152:3 977:83; *Am J Public Health* 1992 82:10 1380-2; *J Ped* 1995 127:5 691-9 – smoking in pregnancy and infant health, with particular reference to Sudden Infant Death Syndrome and Respiratory Illnesses; *Am J Public Health* 1994 84:7 1127-31 – smoking and low birth weight, intrauterine growth retardation; *BMJ* 1995 311 531-6 – smoking and prematurity; *BMJ* 1994 308 1473-6; *Am J Public Health* 1996 86:2 249-53 – smoking and congenital defects.

Am J Public Health 1992 82, 85, 87, 91 – smoking, alcohol and caffeine interactions.

Effects of Smoking on the Fetus, Neonate and Child D. Poswillo and E. Alberman (OUP) 1992; *The Health Benefits of Smoking Cessation: A Report of the Surgeon General* (US Dept Health and Human Services) 1990 – smoking and fertility.

'Fertility and Smoking' *Lancet* 1992 reference.

BMJ 1991, *British Journal General Practice*; *BMJ* 1995, *Am J Public Health* 1994, reference for Canadian/Montreal study.

JAMA 1991 226:22 3174-7 – Nicotine replacement therapies and pregnancy.

Chapter 14

Obs Gyn 1988 72:4 541-4; on amphetamine use in pregnancy.

Neurotoxicol - Teratol 1987 Jan-Feb 9:1 1-7; *Neurobehav-Toxical-Teratol* 1984 Sept-Oct 6:5 345-50; *Am J Obs Gyn* 1984 150:1 23-7; on cannabis use in pregnancy.

Obs Gyn 1989 73-2 157-60; *Am J Perinatal* 1988 5:3 206-7; *J Pediatr* 1988 113:2 354-8; *Teratology* 1988 37:3 201-4; *Neurotoxicol-Teratol* 1987 9:4 291-3; *J Pediatr* 1987 110:1 93-6; for the effects of cocaine on mothers and babies.

Arch Dis Childhood 1988 Jan 63:1 81-3; *Br J Clin Res* 1986 Sept 20 293: 6549; *Neurobehav-Toxicol-Teratol* 1986 Jul-Aug 8:4 357-62; for the harmful effects of heroin in pregnancy.

Adict behav 1988 13:1 275-83; *Obs Gyn* 1988 71:3 ptl 399-404; *Neuro-behav-Toxocol-Teratol* 1984 Jul-Aug 6:4 271-5; *Am J Drug-Alcohol-Abuse* 1984 10:2 195-207; for the effects of methadone in pregnancy.

Teratology 1972 6:75-90; for LSD in pregnancy.

Child Abuse Neglect 1986 10:41-4; *Pediatrics* 1980 65:18-20; for the effects of phencyclidine in pregnancy.

Obs Gyn 1988 71:5 715-8; for solvent abuse in pregnancy.

Pregnancy, Drugs and Smoking J. Hawksley (Franklin Watts/ Gloucester) 1989; *The Pregnant Drug Addict* C. Siney (Books for Midwives Press) 1995; *Drugs, Pregnancy and Childcare* (Institute for the Study of Drug Dependency) 1995; The Effects of Prenatal Exposure of Marijuana, Cocaine, Heroin and Methadone N. Day et al in *Prenatal Exposure to Toxicants: Developmental Consequences* H. Needleman ed John Hopkins 1994; *Int J Gyn Obs* 1994 47:1 73-80; *Substance Abuse in Pregnancy* W. Chawkin Chapter 13 in *Reproductive Health Care for Women and Babies* B. Sachs ed (OUP) 1995; *Drugs in Pregnancy and Lactation: a Reference Guide to Fetal and Neonatal Risk* G. Briggs (Williams and Wilkins) 1994; *Am J Public Health* 1993 83:suppl – for an overview of illegal drug use and effects in pregnancy.

Br J Hosp Med 1993 49:1 51-5 – on increasing drug use; *J Drug Educ* 1992 22:1 15-24 – on attitudes.

Acta Paed 1996 85:2 204-8 – on effects of amphetamine use in pregnancy on longer term child development.

Child Abuse J Bays (Balliere Tyndall) 1993 121-47; *NEJM* 1989 320 762-8; *Adoption & Fostering* 1989 13:4 42-4 – on effects of cannabis.

Obs Gyn 1991 77:4 504-9; *J Obs Gyn* 1988 71:5 715-8 – on solvent abuse and pregnancy.

J Urol 1990 144:1 110-12; *Am J Perinat* 1995 12:6 425-8; *Am J Obs Gyn* 1994 171:6 1556-9 – on cocaine and congenital renal abnormalities; *Pediatrics* 1992 89:6 1199-1203; 1995 95:4 539-45; 1995 96:6 1070-7 - on effects of cocaine on infant behaviour; *Arch Ped Adorsc Med* 1994 148:11 1163-9; *J Ped* 1993 122:6 945-9 – cocaine and congenital heart problems; *Am J Obs Gyn* 1994 171:2 372-9 – on dangers of occasional use of cocaine.

Add to effects of cocaine list: *Pediatrics* 1992 89:2 284-9.

Druglink 1994 July/August 13 – on heroin and pregnancy.

Current Obs Gyn 1993 3 54-8 – on management of withdrawal.

Chapter 15

A Practical Guide to Labour Management D. Gibb (Blackwell Scientific Publications) 1988; The Management of Labour ed J. Studd (Black-well Scientific Publications) 1985; *Br J Obs Gyn* 1982 89:4; for the usefulness and frequency of induction.

Obs Gyn 1986 67:1 21-4; *World Med* 1983 Sep p. 215; *Ob Gyn News* 1985 20:10 15-31; on nipple stimulation.

The Assertive Pregnancy N. Wesson (Grapevine) 1987; on acupuncture.

Am J Obs Gyn 1989 160:3 529-35; *J Obs Gyn* 1988 8:suppl s7-s11; *Midwife HV Commun Nurse* 1987 23:1 12-7; for the advantages and disadvantages of prostaglandins.

Active Management of Labour K. O'Driscoll and D. Meagher (Saunders) 1980; *J Obs Gyn* 1988 158:2 255-8; for the arguments in favour of active management.

Birth 1988 15:4 199-202; *Lancet* 1988 1:8581 p. 352; *Obs Gyn* 1988 71:2 150-4; *J Obs Gyn* 1988 8:Suppl 16-7; for the pros and cons of induction and acceleration with oxytocin.

Lancet May 1, 1982 p. 991-4; on jaundice following oxytocin.

Chapter 16
Birth 1985 12:4 205-13; for women's feelings about epidurals.

Science 1979 204: 391-2 and 205; 474-8; *Clin Obs Gyn* 1981 24:2 649-69; for drug effects on the baby.

A Guide to Effective Care in Pregnancy and Childbirth M. Enkin (OUP) 2nd edition 1995.

Who's Having Your Baby? B. Beech (AIMS), *Drugs in Labour and Birth*, D. Maire (AIMS).

Chapter 17
'Use of pethidine in labour' an Information Sheet published by the National Childbirth Trust (see page 209), 1989; *Aust J Adv Nursing* 1986 4:1 13-189; *Clin Pharm* 1986 11:4 283-98; *Am J Obs Gyn* 1985 51:3 406-9; *Obs Gyn* 1984 64:5 724-7; for information on pethidine.

Acta Obs Gyn Scand 1984 63:7617-9; for the effects of naloxone.

Am J Perinatal 1988 5:3 197-200; *J Perinatal Med* 1986 14:2 131 *Clin Pharmacokinet* 1986 11:4 28398; *Percept Mot Skills* 1984 58:3 859-66; *Acta Obst Gyn Scand* 1983 62:6 549-53; *Br J Obs Gyn* 1983 90:1 28-33; for the effects of pethidine on the baby.

Anaesth 1987 42:1 7-14; *Postgrad Med J* 1985 61:supp 2 23-6; for the effects of Meptid.

Clin Pharm 1986 11:4 283-98; for the effects of nitrous oxide.

'Some Women's Experience with Epidurals' S. Kitzinger published by National Childbirth Trust (see page 209) 1987; *Midwifery* 1985 1:32-6; *BMJ* 11 Sept 1982 285: 689; *Update* 1 Mar 1986 401-8; *Pain* 1984 pp.321-37; for the effectiveness of epidurals as pain relief.

J Perinatal Med 1986 14:4 239; *Scientific American* 1986 255:4 100-7; *Birth* 1986 13:4 227-40; for the hazards and benefits of stress in labour.

Anaesth 1988 43:2 154-5; on inserting epidurals.

Acta Anaesth Scand 1986 30:7 584-7; *Anaesth Intensive Care* 1986 14:4 412-7; on epidurals and shivering.

Can J Anaesth 1988 35:1 41-6; on epidurals and low blood pressure.

J Obs Gyn 1988 28:1 17-24; on ambulatory epidurals.

European J Obs Gyn Reprod Boil 1989 30:1 27-33; *J Am Board Fam Pract* 1088 1:14 238-44; *J Obs Gyn* 1988 9:2 122-5; *Obs Gyn* 1987 69:5 770-3; for the effects of epidurals on the second stage of labour.

BMJ 1989 23 Sept 751-2; *Can J Anaesth* 1987 34:3 ptl 294-9; *Anaesthesia* 1986 41:12 1240-50; *Obs Gyn* 1985 65:6 837-9; on hazards of epidurals.

Acta Anaesth Scand 1987 31:4 347-51; 'Behavioural Teratology' in *Perinatal Epidemiology* ed M. Bracken (Oxford University Press) 1984; *Br J Obs Gyn* 1981 88:4 407-13; for the effects of epidurals on the baby.
Pain Relief in Childbirth N. Bradford and Chamberlain (HarperCollins) 1995 – general information.
Modern Midwife 1995 5:1 8-11 – on acupuncture for labour pain.

Chapter 18
BMJ 1988 Nov 19 297:6659 1295-300; *Midwives Chron* 1989 102:1215 130; *Birthrights* S. Inch (Hutchinson)1982; for the arguments for and against syntometrine use.
Can Med Asso J 1988 139:127-30; *NZ Med J* 1988 101:507-8; *Midwifery* 1987 3:4 170-7; on Vitamin K for the baby.
Anaes 1992 48:1 63-5 – on use of epidurals, *Int J Obs Anaesth* 1995 4:3 133-9; *Birth* 1994 2:3 172-4; *BMJ* 1990 301 9-12; *BJM* 1992 304 1279-82; *BMJ* 1993 306 1299-303; *Int J Obs Anaes* 1995 4:1 21-5 – on complications and longer term effects of epidurals with particular reference to backache; *Lancet* 1993 344:8931 1238 – on patient controlled epidural.

Chapter 19
A Guide to Effective Care in Pregnancy and Childbirth M. Enkin (OUP) 2nd edition, 1995.
Delivering your Placenta – the Third Stage (AIMS).

Index